FEEDING
THE YOUNG Athlete

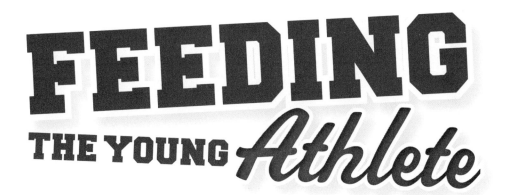

FEEDING
THE YOUNG *Athlete*

SPORTS NUTRITION MADE EASY
FOR PLAYERS, PARENTS AND COACHES

CYNTHIA LAIR WITH **SCOTT MURDOCH**, Ph.D., RD

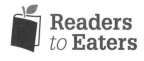

Readers *to* Eaters

Bellevue, Washington

The information in this book has been prepared thoughtfully and carefully.
It is not intended to be diagnostic or prescriptive. Any athlete, young or old, should have
regular physical examinations by his or her health-care practitioner.

READERS to EATERS Books
12437 SE 26th Place
Bellevue, WA 98005
Distributed by Publishers Group West

www.ReadersToEaters.com

Printed in the U.S.A. by Worzalla, Stevens Point, Wisconsin (8/12)

Book design by Red Herring Design
Book production by The Kids at Our House

10 9 8 7 6 5 4 3 2 1
Second Edition

Cataloging-in-Publication data is on file at the Library of Congress
ISBN 978-0-9836615-2-8

READERS to EATERS Books may be purchased for corporate, educational, or other promotional sales.
For special discounts and information, contact us at Info@ReadersToEaters.com.

Dedications

Here's to the Barracudas, the Crunch, the Momentum, the Braves, the Fusion and the Scots. These strong young women turned me into an avid soccer fan and magnified my education about how food works. —C. L.

To Pat and our two wondrous boys, who continually inspire me to spend my time and energy mindfully on those pursuits that matter most. —S. M.

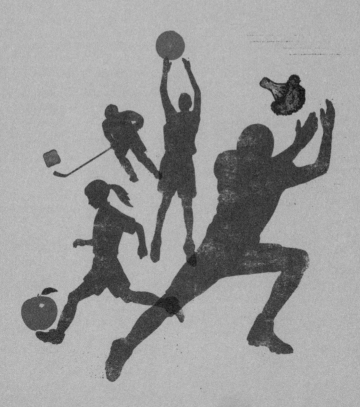

TABLE OF *Contents*

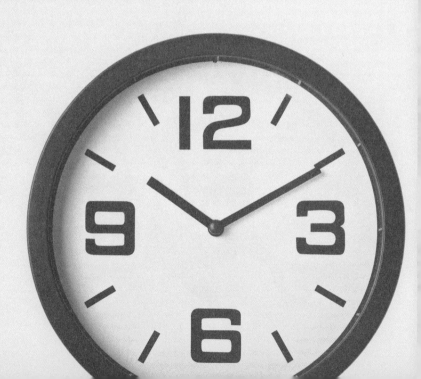

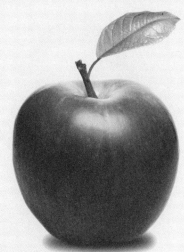

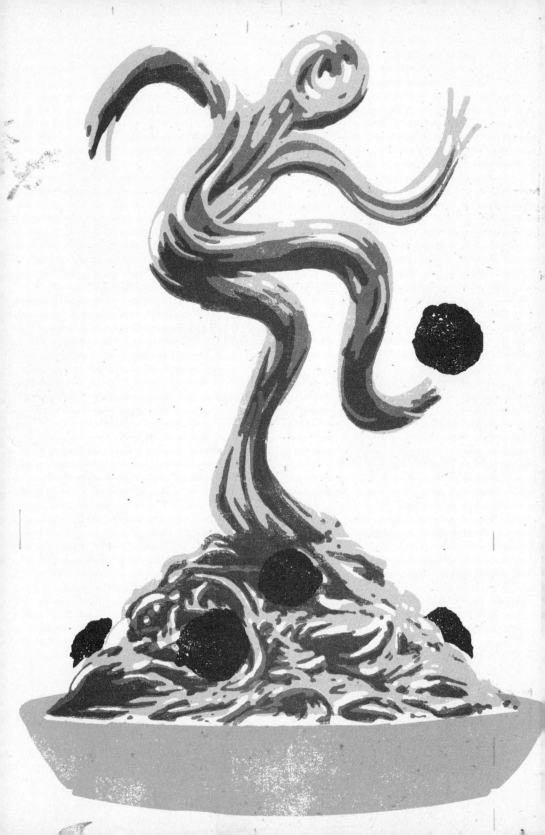

INTRODUCTION

My daughter, Grace, started playing competitive sports when she was seven years old. I had never been involved in sports as a child or an adult, so I found the sports sideline fun and perplexing. Observing the post-game mêlée of packaged junk food flying into the hungry mouths of children disturbed me, especially since I teach family nutrition and cooking with whole foods at a university. As if holidays, birthdays and the kids' menu in restaurants didn't create enough excuses for feeding children poor food, here was yet another excuse for a sugar frenzy. At the very moment when the body needs an intense refueling of nutrient-rich foods, parents unknowingly doled out snacks such as Ding Dongs.

As my daughter became a more skilled player and was selected to be on more competitive teams, she played in tournaments every weekend. So making sure that she had the fuel to maintain her performance became crucial. Not only was I motivated to help my daughter maintain the starting position she wanted, I had also become invested in the whole team. I wanted all the players on the team to be empowered by their food choices.

I sought the help of my colleague, Dr. Scott Murdoch. He has a doctorate in nutrition and human performance and is a Registered Dietitian as well. But more importantly, he was also an athlete who competed in triathlons and professional tennis. Dr. Murdoch is a science nonfiction kind of guy with all sorts of facts, and the research to back them up. I would translate the complex data he gave me into language that could be comprehended by a young athlete or into recipes I could make in my kitchen. Then, I'd try out the food and the timing of eating with my daughter's team.

They won a lot of games.

I was happy to see that with some simple nutrition education, the players on the teams (my daughter played soccer all through middle school, high school and college) began to feel the connection between food and athletic performance. Pumped about sharing what I was learning with players and coaches, I generated handouts and folders, and finally with too many pages to wrangle, this book began to emerge.

Young people who are physically active benefit from better health, confidence and well-being. For activity to be truly healthy and enjoyable, however, children need to eat wholesome foods. Both Dr. Murdoch and I believe that being physically active without eating wholesome foods, or eating wholesome foods without any activity, is simply self-defeating.

There is a huge rise in the number of young people participating in sports, yet there is a dearth of easy-to-understand and practical information on the topic of sports nutrition for kids. Bastyr University, where both Dr. Murdoch and I have taught, is a school on the cutting edge of medicine and nutrition. The nutrition department combines the best of modern scientific research with the wisdom of promoting natural, whole foods. Using our combined backgrounds in exercise physiology, sports nutrition, whole foods cooking and family nutrition, we have created a practical, easy-to-read resource to fill this gap.

In this expanded second edition, we've reorganized our discussion to highlight what to eat, when to eat and how to shop, so players can be mindful about snacks they can pack or food to buy when they're traveling to a distant game. Appreciating the crammed schedules of those who are involved in team sports, we organized the book using lists and key takeaways. Families and teams can grasp at a glance the reasoning behind our guidelines, as well as ways to apply them.

One further addition is that the title now specifies the book as an educational resource for players, parents AND coaches. This had been implied in the first edition but never spelled out. Considering the impact that coaches have on young people, it seemed important to call them to action. When the coach is on board with helping players understand the impact of food on performance, the message is more likely to be heard and practiced.

Although this book is ideal for individuals participating in organized sports, the information is applicable to anyone who has a physically active lifestyle.

While we all feel pressed for time, the push to COOK is less of an undertone and more of a directive in this edition. A small percentage of kids who play sports go on to play in college. An even smaller fraction of those will play professional sports. But I hope young athletes will carry their appreciation for movement into adulthood and also carry forward their knowledge of the relationship between food and the body. Seeing and practicing the skill of cooking increase the likelihood that the food-body relationship will be a positive one.

This is a golden opportunity! Eating well increases energy, endurance and the ability to concentrate, both on and off the field. Players who eat and drink well have an edge over their competition, especially in the second half of the game, the second game of the day or the second half of the season. Educating young players, parents and coaches about sports nutrition offers a gateway to improved performance and lifelong eating habits.

Eat better to play your best!

—Cynthia

PART ONE

HOW TO COACH YOUNG ATHLETES

Plan ahead.
Timing is everything.
Strive for wholeness.

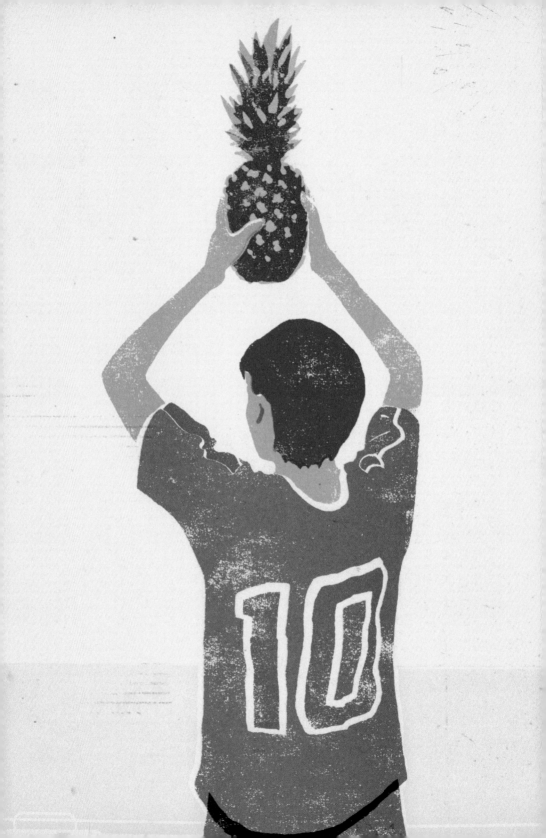

1

The Ten Essential Eating Guidelines for Superb Performance

Do This

Wise up to how foods create energy

Eat using the timetable

Sip, sip, sip

Supercharge with whole grains

Chomp fruits and vegetables

Put protein in its place

Sideline the sugar

Make your plate whole

Relax, recover, rebuild

Get the whole team involved

Everyone can benefit from understanding the basic science behind how food works. But when young people involved in sports apply them, the advantages can be surprisingly immediate. Here are ten simple guidelines for improving and sustaining athletic performance. Get down with these positive strategies and find a new groove to your game.

WISE UP TO HOW FOODS CREATE ENERGY

Nature designed foods to form a team of nutrients

The main nutritional components of foods are carbohydrates, proteins, fats, vitamins, minerals, fiber and water. Each nutrient has a specific purpose in the body.

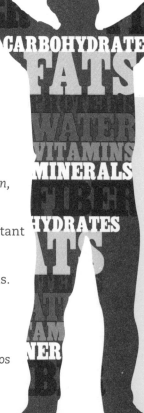

Carbohydrates are used to create energy. Foods that contain carbohydrates work the quickest to transform into muscle glycogen—primary fuel for muscles. *Sources: whole grain bread, brown rice, oatmeal, corn tortillas, quinoa*

Proteins promote cell growth and repair, and regulate many body processes such as water balancing, nutrient transport and muscle contraction. *Sources: eggs, fish, chicken, turkey, beef, cheese, beans*

Fats transport a variety of important nutrients like vitamins A and D, and are a major component of cell walls. Fats are also used as a slow, secondary energy source. *Sources: butter, olive oil, nuts and seeds, nut butters, avocados*

Vitamins keep body processes working properly. They play a key role in transforming carbohydrates into glycogen. *Sources: dark leafy greens, sweet potatoes, strawberries, oranges*

Minerals provide essential materials for the athletic body. For example, calcium and magnesium are used for bone development, and iron for oxygen transport. *Sources: dark leafy greens, sea vegetables (like nori), dairy, bananas*

Fiber helps food move through the body while promoting healthy bacteria in the gastro-intestinal tract.

Fiber helps bodies feel full and satisfied with the right amount of calories.

Sources: whole grains, beans, fruits, vegetables

Water constitutes the majority of our body weight, anywhere from 55% to 65%. Dehydration impairs all bodily functions, including brains and muscles. *Sources: water, ice chips, Homemade Sports Drink (page 70)*

NUTRIENTS WORK TOGETHER LIKE A TEAM

Just as it's more effective to play basketball with a whole team rather than one player, nutrients work more efficiently when they are matched up with the right teammates.

A good example is the nutrient calcium. If you take a pill that is 100% calcium and nothing else, it's on the field alone. But if the calcium has the right amount of other team players like magnesium and vitamin C, the calcium will perform at its highest level and your body will absorb more of the nutrients. This is called bioavailability.

Nature creates WHOLE foods

A food from nature doesn't have just one nutrient, but a group of them. An apple has carbohydrates, fiber, vitamins, minerals and water. Whole foods are nutrient-rich, meaning they have a whole bunch of great players on a team. Just like players on the field, every nutrient has its purpose. Once you understand what it is, you can create a winning game plan. And if you realize that eating whole foods ensures the meal is full of the nutrients your body needs to play well—you're halfway to home plate.

Before we put a bite in our mouths, we need to take a moment to consider where the food came from. What was its life like before it came to be on the grocery store shelf? Foods that are in packages can be pretty mysterious.

Get in the habit of reading labels. If it's a whole food, you should be able to recognize every ingredient as something that grows in nature.

How to tell if a food is a WHOLE food

Consider these questions when choosing foods that are worthy of putting in your body.

Does it grow in nature?
It's easy to imagine carrots growing in the ground or an apple on a tree, but not so easy to picture where Twinkies might "grow." The pale green color of an avocado illustrates nature's magic, whereas the "arctic" blue coloring in a beverage does not have natural origins.

How many ingredients does it have?
Most whole foods have only ONE ingredient. Foods like bananas, salmon or green beans don't need labels. They are whole foods from nature. Count how many ingredients are listed on most packaged foods!

What's been done to the food since it was harvested?
Imagine how the food was made and what was done to it before it arrived at the grocery store. The less the food is processed, the more likely it is a WHOLE food. Packaged foods that have long ingredient lists with hard-to-pronounce ingredient names likely have had their "wholeness" compromised.

Are all the edible parts of the food present?

Juice is only part of a fruit. Oil is only part of the olive. White rice is missing its outer hull that is full of fiber and nutrients. When you eat un-whole foods, your body in its natural wisdom will crave the parts it didn't get.

Could you make this food in your kitchen?

An example of something you can't make in your kitchen is soy protein isolate. In contrast, tofu is a traditional soy food that has been made in Asian home kitchens for centuries. Soy protein isolate is a complex refined food, while tofu is a simple food made from cooked, strained and coagulated soybeans. A good litmus test is to ask yourself if what you're eating is something that could be made in a kitchen.

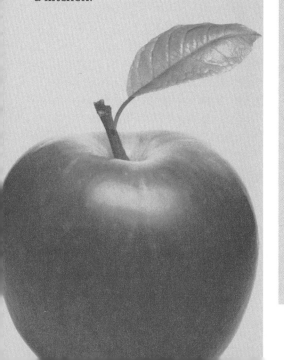

3

THREE BIG REASONS TO EAT WHOLE FOODS

You **know** what you're eating – food made by nature, not in a factory

Whole foods have a **team** of nutrients to help you create energy, not just one

You'll feel more **energized** because your body is not wasting energy trying to decide how to store or dispose of non-food ingredients that may be added to packaged foods

Don't be fooled by labels

Big flashy words on labels grab our attention. Packaged foods designed to entice athletes use lots of Batman terms: "Kapow!" "Zing!" "Power!" "Hammer." "Crunch." These food labels also promise to "build muscle," "increase endurance," "boost energy," "protect muscles" and so on. Smart athletes look beyond the dazzle and hunt for the list of ingredients on the back of packages. Now we're talking.

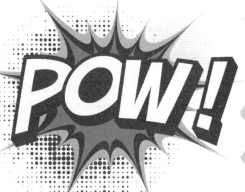

Students in my nutrition class will often hold up a bar or drink and ask me, "Is this okay?" I never give a straight yes or no. Instead, I ask them, "What's in it?" As they read the ingredient list, I may interrupt and ask, "What's THAT?" When they shrug, I encourage them to look it up. They may reply, "But the label says it's good for you!" Yes, indeed. Exactly what the food manufacturer wants you to believe!

Shoppers often believe what they read on food labels and pay the price for foods that have been altered and enhanced with a very long ingredient list. Do you recognize all of the ingredients? Are they whole foods or isolates? (Isolates are identifiable by their scientific names.) What are the first three ingredients?

Ingredients are listed in the order of greatest to least amount in a food product. If one or more of the first three ingredients are sugar and/or a form of sugar (words that end with the letters -ose), don't add the packaged food to your cart. Stay aware.

! Know what you're putting into your body

These two snacks have about the same number of calories and cost relatively the same if the sandwich is made with organic ingredients. But you're paying for things you may not want in your body when you buy the "Way Past Crazy" bar. Notice that the main ingredient in the bar, disguised by the name "4X Energy Fusion," is just sugar, sugar, sugar and sugar.

Example 1
"Way Past Crazy" bar

Ingredient list: 4X Energy Fusion blend (organic evaporated cane juice syrup, maltodextrin, fructose, dextrose), oat bran, soy protein isolate, alkalized cocoa, brown rice flour, and 2% or less of canola oil, vegetable glycerin, salt, chocolate, natural flavor, nonfat milk, almond butter, peanut flour. Minerals: calcium phosphate, potassium phosphate, ferrous fumarate (iron). Vitamins: ascorbic acid (vitamin C), vitamin B6 hydrochloride, riboflavin (vitamin B2), thiamine mononitrate (vitamin B1).

Example 2
Stayin' Sane PB & B sandwich

Recipe: Spread a tablespoon of peanut butter on a slice of 100% whole wheat bread (whole wheat flour, water, yeast, honey, salt). Top with banana slices. Eat open-faced or folded over.

EAT USING THE TIMETABLE

Schedule when and what to eat before, during and after an athletic event

My daughter, Grace, played on a select soccer team when she was in middle school. Another girl, Allison, was a talented center-mid on the team and a head taller than most girls her age. Needless to say, she was an important part of the winning team. One day, Allison arrived on the field after the warm-up for an early morning game. As she was crossing the field and pulling on her cleats, her mother came chasing behind, waving a bagel and yelling, "Here! HERE! You've got to eat something."

A bagel made of white flour was not the best or worst choice, but the timing was awful. There was not a chance that Allison would have the fuel needed to play a strong first half. Even if she had eaten the bagel as she shoved on her shin guards, there just wasn't enough time for her body to transform the food into muscle energy, or glycogen.

Why the pre-game meal is so important

Glycogen is made from the foods we eat (particularly carbohydrate-containing foods) and is stored inside each of our muscle fibers to provide muscles with fuel. However, muscles can only store a limited amount of glycogen at a time, so we must constantly replenish our stores by eating.

It is critical to eat a healthy meal containing ample carbohydrates prior to a game or practice in order to have the muscle energy to play at your full potential. Never come to a game, practice or scrimmage without fuel in the tank. When our glycogen levels are low we become slower, weaker and less able to concentrate.

When is game time? Check out the timetable on page 28 and plan ahead when and what to eat.

! Eat two to three hours before ● your game

Some players try to down an energy bar or a piece of toast right before the game because they didn't eat anything earlier. If you do this, the food will sit uncomfortably undigested in your stomach.

When I lecture on this topic to teams, I will ask if any of them has ever gone without breakfast and lunch. I usually get a few hands up. Then I ask, "How did you feel?" Without hesitation they say, "Spaced out."

The first thing to suffer when you haven't eaten is not the muscle in your legs, but the big "muscle" in your head—the brain.

Quick decision-making becomes impossible. This paves the way for not only poor performance, but also injuries.

Top the tank at half-time and breaks

If you have quick metabolism or tend to drag during the second half of the game, consider a half-time snack to help maintain energy throughout the game. Plan ahead and be prepared. The best snack choice is a fruit with high water content: oranges, tangerines, melons, grapes and pineapple rings. These will give you some fast-acting carbohydrates and hydration with every bite.

Don't try out new half-time snacks for the first time at a game. Bring a fruit to practice and eat it during the break. Then see if it is helpful or not. Did you feel your energy pick up? If it did, and you "stomached" it well, then you can try the half-time snack at the next game.

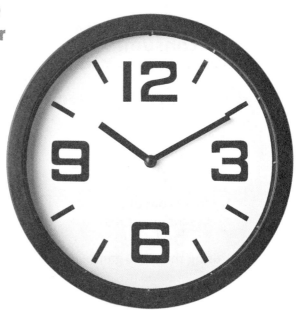

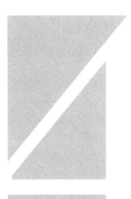

Take advantage of opportunities to restore yourself. When you come off the field for substitution, during time-outs for injuries or at half-time, drink fluids and, if needed, eat a juicy whole fruit.

Refuel quickly to come back stronger

Research has shown that our muscles are able to replenish glycogen needs more quickly when we eat or drink carbohydrate-containing foods within the first 30 minutes after a game or practice. During this time, muscles will convert carbohydrates into glycogen up to three times faster than if you wait and eat two hours after the game. This is your glycogen window.

Take advantage of the glycogen window and eat healthy carbohydrate-rich snacks and beverages as soon as you can after the game or practice has finished.

This snack or meal is extremely important if you have another game, scrimmage or practice within 12 to 24 hours. Ideally, if you have a second game on the same day, you will have a small nutritious snack immediately after the first game,

FOUR BIG WAYS TO TOP THE TANK AT HALFTIME

When you come off the field **consume** fluids and carbohydrates

Whole, juicy **fruits** work best

Water with ¼ cup of lemonade or fruit juice also works

Try snacks out at practice or scrimmage first **before** using them in a game followed by a more substantial meal after the second game.

Circumstances don't always allow for optimal sports nutrition. If someone forgot to bring snacks or there's no time to stop and get something to eat, don't panic. Recovery is attainable later; it's just that the body is more efficient immediately after the event. Another thing to remember is that calories of any kind consumed post-game are better than no calories at all.

Note what time your game, event or practice starts and work backward

If the game starts at 10:00 a.m., be sure that you get up early enough to eat breakfast by 8:00 a.m. If you don't have gas in the tank, the car can't go. If you don't eat at the right time, your muscles won't have fuel for practice or the game. Any deficit you experience today will make it even more difficult to replenish the next day.

You may be thinking, "I just can't eat that early in the morning," or, "I can do fine with soda and an energy bar." If you've ever had those thoughts, change the way you think. You're not Superman, the Incredible Hulk or any

When you pack your sports bag for the game, be sure to include an extra piece of fruit, sandwich or muffin—some kind of snack.

Make it part of the pre-game ritual before you leave the house. This way you'll be less likely to miss the window.

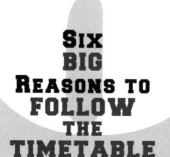

SIX BIG REASONS TO FOLLOW THE TIMETABLE

Dramatically increases **stamina** to last the whole game

Increases mental **focus** to play strategically

Helps maintain **performance** levels game after game

Aids in **recovery** from games and practices

Helps **prevent** performance **slumps**

Helps **prevent injury**

kind of Hornet. You are flesh and blood, requiring food to live, and good food to perform well.

Low muscle glycogen is directly related to fatigue, decreased running speed, slow thinking and poor recovery.

The timing and choices in the athlete's diet are the most fixable aspect of improving performance...and often the most overlooked.

For early-morning games, start eating the evening before

Eat an excellent pre-game dinner the night before. See pre-game meal ideas in Chapter 8 (page 105). While not generally recommended, having a snack an hour before going to bed can be helpful. See post-game snack ideas in Chapters 6 & 7 (pages 87 & 101). No candy, soda or ice cream the night before competition. Have a pre-game snack or mini-breakfast one to two hours before the game.

 This pre-game snack is very important

3 EARLY MORNING PRE-GAME SNACKS

1

Half a whole grain bagel, muffin, scone or toast
(not a sweet roll or doughnut)

2

Small amount of yogurt and/or a piece of fruit

3

Big glass of water

Don't forget to eat before and after practice

Many parents and players get serious about eating and drinking when a game or competition is at stake. It is equally important to remember to hydrate and fuel up before and after every practice or training session. All too often, practices are held during after-school hours, long after lunch.

If you haven't eaten since lunch-time, you will need a hearty snack or mini-meal and water before heading out the door. Keep in mind that how you eat today affects how you play tomorrow. Inadequate intake on training days can make it nearly impossible to fuel optimally on game days.

And, take your time

Remember to CHEW! Don't wolf down food. Your stomach will have to do the work if your teeth don't. You can eat a very nutrient-rich meal, but if you don't absorb the nutrients due to poor digestion, you won't benefit from eating. Good absorption requires eating food in an unhurried manner. Eating in the company of friends, in a relaxed atmosphere, enhances digestion.

CHEW!

TIMETABLE TO PLAY YOUR BEST GAME

2-3 hours before a game	**EAT A PRE-GAME MEAL** A pre-game plate of pasta, rice, bread or potatoes AND vegetables, PLUS some protein. **Don't stuff yourself.**	**DRINK FLUIDS** .5 – 1 liter 
1-2 hours before a game	**EAT A PRE-GAME SNACK** Fresh fruit, crackers, bread, energy bar (read the label first!) **Very light fare, if needed.**	**DRINK FLUIDS** .5 – 1 liter
0-1 hour before a game	# NO FOOD	**DRINK FLUIDS** .5 – 1 liter
Game time (or training)	**EAT A HALF-TIME JUICY FRUIT** Fruit with high water content, orange or melon slices, grapes **Optional, if needed.**	**DRINK FLUIDS WITH CARBS** .5 – 1 liter
0-1 hour after a game	**EAT A POST-GAME SNACK** 100% fruit juice, fresh fruit, bagel, muffin, sandwich, crackers, energy bars, liquid meals **Any snack is better than no snack.**	**DRINK FLUIDS** 2 liters over several hours

SIP, SIP, SIP

Hydration needs to happen before, during and after exertion

Before a game or practice, drink at least a half liter spread out over an hour and a half.

Drink a glass of water before the pre-game meal. Keep filled water bottles by the door so that grabbing one on the way to the car is easy to remember. Sip from the water bottle in the car on the way to the game. It's more effective to sip water than to chug it down. If you try to down two cups of water in one sitting, you may end up with a sloshing belly and be too bloated to play your best.

At the game venue, continue sipping a minimum of a half liter.

Often players are nervous, busy practicing drills or just being silly with the energy of having friends and teammates around, and they forget to drink. Drinking at this point is even more critical when playing in hot weather. Parents and coaches can set a good example by bringing water bottles and drinking frequently, too.

During time-outs and half-times, continue sipping at least a half liter.

Parents and coaches can be helpful by calling out reminders such as, "Drink ten sips before you go back in," or "Eight big swigs and then let's talk about the second half." Parents need to make sure there is always water available on the sideline so no one goes without. Perhaps the team can designate a parent to bring water to every game.

Post-game rehydration means sipping two liters over several hours.

Parents can hand out water after the game to ensure post-game hydration. Drinking water after play helps the body flush out waste so that recovery is quicker. Without appropriate amounts of liquid, you may feel more sluggish and tired after an event. This can become quite a hindrance during tournaments when there is more than one game or event per day.

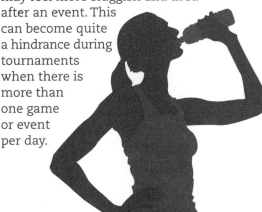

How much to drink depends on you and the conditions

Some players may require more water, some a bit less. Hydration is more crucial in a strenuous game such as soccer than it is for a less aerobic sport such as softball. Hot weather or even a stuffy gym will demand more frequent hydration.

If you are serious about priming for an event, simple hydration tests provide important feedback. A practical way to gauge how much water you need to drink is to check your urine color—when it runs clear, you're adequately hydrated. Coaches and parents can remind players to "drink until you pee clear." At one team nutrition seminar, we counted how many sips it took each player to finish half a cup of fluid. That way each player knew exactly how many swallows constituted a cup.

Staying hydrated is especially important for prepubescent athletes, since they don't sweat as much as adults and have higher metabolic rates than adults.

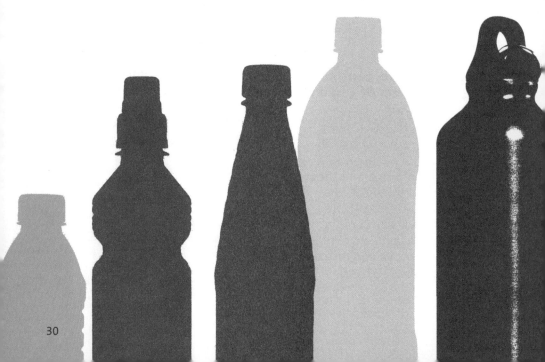

! It's important to drink even if you ● don't feel thirsty

Sometimes during vigorous exercise your sense of thirst is NOT engaged, yet you must continue to hydrate to regulate body temperature and eliminate metabolic waste. It is not necessary to drink pre-formulated drinks. These drinks may be convenient, but they're expensive and won't give you more or better nutrients than an apple, some grape juice, or a bagel sandwich. See "Drink This" and "Don't Drink This" in Chapter 4 (page 65).

THREE BIG REASONS TO HYDRATE

Hydration is crucial for proper **muscle functioning**

Hydration is key for **quick thinking—** our brains are 90% water

Hydration is needed to **regulate body temperature** and eliminate waste

SUPERCHARGE WITH WHOLE GRAINS

Eating carbohydrates is the most efficient way to make glycogen

Ethiopian runners attribute their dominance in long-distance races in part to their diet, which includes the whole grain teff, an easily absorbed complex carbohydrate with appreciable amounts of protein, calcium and iron.

When you eat starchy foods like teff or brown rice, the carbohydrates are converted into blood sugar (or glucose), which muscles and the brain use for energy. Any glucose that's not immediately used is stored in the muscles and liver as glycogen, which is the preferred fuel for muscles working at moderate to high intensities.

When glycogen levels are low, the body begins the inefficient method of making glucose from protein and fat. This conversion of protein and fat to glucose can't keep up with your energy needs during games or practice. Another side effect of inadequate carbohydrate intake is impaired central nervous system function—that spacey feeling experienced when you skip a meal.

Carbohydrates need teammates—vitamins and minerals and some protein—to make glycogen. Whole grains are an excellent source of carbohydrates because they contain more nutrients than refined grains. In addition to carbohydrates, whole grains contain vitamins and minerals, some protein and fat, and fiber, while refined grains such as white flour or white rice only contain carbohydrates. Nothing else.

! Eat foods rich in carbohydrates pre-game

So when planning pre-game meals, put carbohydrates in the form of whole grains front and center. But don't forget to include fresh fruits, vegetables and some protein as teammates.

12 SUPERCHARGING WHOLE GRAINS

1 Brown Rice
Unmilled whole grain with hull, bran and germ

2 Bulgur
A quick cooking whole wheat

3 Corn
Indigenous grain of Americas

4 Kasha
Toasted buckwheat groats

5 Millet
Indigenous grain of Asia

6 Steel-cut Oats
Thinly sliced whole oats

7 Polenta
Italian cornmeal

8 Quinoa
Ancient grain of Peru

9 Soba
Japanese noodles made from buckwheat flour

10 Teff
Ancient grain of Ethiopia

11 Whole Wheat
Unrefined whole grain with bran and germ

12 Wild Rice
Indigenous grain of Americas

CHOMP FRUITS AND VEGETABLES

Fruits and vegetables provide nutrients to convert food into what your body needs

The most reliable source of vitamins and minerals is fresh vegetables and fruit. By fruits and vegetables, we mean whole, recognizable foods like apples, oranges, broccoli and spinach. Fruit leather, juices and boxed cereal with fruity bits don't count.

It takes extensive processing and refining in a factory to strip a whole food of its vitamins and minerals. Yet, many of the products on our grocery store shelves are canned, boxed, frozen, lifeless foods that have been robbed of vital nutrients. Walk on by.

! Set your sights on the produce aisle

Colorful fruits and vegetables enrich your athletic body while salty junk food and sugary treats deplete it.

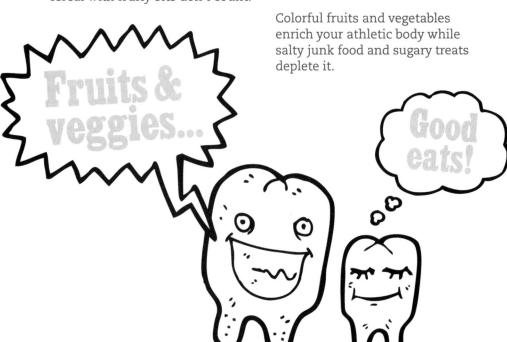

Fruits & veggies...

Good eats!

Fresh fruits and vegetables boost the immune system, and keep skin clear and eyes bright. They contain enzymes, antioxidants and hundreds of unique phytonutrients that are essential for optimal health.

Fruits and vegetables are also high in fiber, so they fill you up and satisfy you more quickly than refined foods. Along with protein, they are critical in helping convert carbohydrates into glycogen for your muscles and brain.

More than a quarter of your pre-game meal should be vegetables and fruit.

So don't leave home without them. Always pack a fruit or a container of vegetables in your sports bag. Eating fruits with high water content, such as grapes, oranges and melon, gives you a nice mid-game lift. Fruits and vegetables are also a delicious choice for post-game snacks.

THREE BIG REASONS TO CHOMP FRUITS AND VEGETABLES

They stoke the body with **nutrients** needed to convert food into energy

Deep-colored produce is rich in **phytonutrients** and **antioxidants** that protect your cells from damage

Calcium and other minerals found in dark leafy greens are more bioavailable

PUT PROTEIN IN ITS PLACE

Do not glorify protein by believing more is better

Skip the protein and just go for the carbs? Not smart. Shun the pasta and man-up with an eight-ounce steak? Also not smart. Protein makes hair, skin, organs and muscles grow. The amino acids that make up protein also encourage muscles to become stronger and more efficient, and stimulate the conversion of carbohydrates into muscle glycogen (the type of energy your muscles prefer for fuel). So, no way do you want to leave out the protein from your sports nutrition program.

Hang on. What are amino acids? Well, when you dine on protein, like a roasted chicken leg, the food is broken down into amino acids with funny names like phenylalanine. There are eight essential ones—a cool thing to know because vegetarian players need to combine certain foods to make sure they get all eight in their diet. Most grains lack lysine and most beans are missing methionine, but together they make a complete pair. Keep in mind that protein can't be stored. Eating more than is needed causes the body to expend lots of energy processing it, resulting in the creation of urea, a potent waste product that needs to be excreted via urine. You lose energy and water—two valuable commodities for athletes.

Do athletes need to eat more protein?

Despite the fact that the average American diet far exceeds the recommendations for daily intake of protein, many athletes believe that additional protein will help build muscle and make them stronger. Muscles are made mostly

Experts agree that four to six ounces of protein a day (an amount about the size of your fist) is ample.

of protein, so it seems sensible to believe that the more protein, the more muscle. For elite adult athletes or body builders, there may be some benefit to eating a little more protein. Even for muscle-building adults the advantages plateau at intake levels well below protein amounts consumed by most athletes.

There's no end to the hype around protein powders and their importance to athletes.

If you take a closer look, you'll see that the push for protein supplements comes from marketers who play off the athlete's desire to be competitive.

Most protein supplements add calories as well as protein. Many protein powders contain artificial sweeteners and chemicals that bodies are better off without.

Experts agree that four to six ounces of protein a day (an amount about the size of your fist) is ample. Most Americans eat at least twice that much. For pre- and post-game meals, rely on carbohydrates and foods rich in vitamins and minerals for energy. Include foods containing protein and fat, but in a smaller proportion…no more than a quarter of your plate. Translation: A lot of brown rice and vegetables with some teriyaki chicken strips thrown in.

FOUR BIG WAYS TO PUT PROTEIN IN ITS PLACE

Protein should be **15%** to **25%** of the pre-game meal

Eat larger portions of protein on **non-game** days

Get your protein from **whole foods**: animal (eggs, fish, poultry, meat); vegetarian (dairy); and vegan (nuts, seeds, beans, grains)

Skip the protein powders, protein bars and protein drinks

SIDELINE THE SUGAR

Sugar doesn't supercharge you

When my daughter was playing on the Fusion soccer team in high school, the team counted on a super-duper forward named Jenny. One cool autumn morning just before the game, I heard Jenny tell her teammates that she had a cola and a doughnut for breakfast. She even bragged that she was supercharged and ready to go. The sugar high was apparent as she busted onto the field and darted around for about 15 minutes. Then, abruptly, she asked to come out, saying she was not feeling well and was suddenly tired.

Sugar gives most people a rush of very short-lived energy.

The calories in highly sugared products are empty, or naked.

This means they have no other nutrients associated with them, just simple carbohydrates. Products made with loads of sugar generally contain little protein, fat, fiber, water, vitamins or minerals. They have no teammates. When you eat sugary foods, your body needs the help of other nutrients to process the sugar.

Sugar is refined to such a degree that it doesn't have to go through the normal slow digestive process of breaking down foods in your stomach and intestines. Sugar goes right into your bloodstream. In most cases, this quick entry causes blood glucose levels to shoot up, giving you a rush of frenetic energy. But this feeling of energy doesn't last long.

The body quickly tries to regain its balance, using important nutrients such as B vitamins, calcium, phosphorus, iron, chromium, zinc and manganese to stabilize blood glucose levels. These nutrients are all associated with healthy mental and emotional function and good bone health. What could be more vital to young athletes than excellent concentration, steady composure and strong bones? Yet, so many players come to games fueled up solely on sugary cereals or sweet snacks.

You need a steady source of fuel to get through an athletic event as well as the other "events" taking place in your daily life. Although sugary foods can provide a quick jolt of energy, the biological cost is too high.

Reconsider sugary rewards after working so hard

We have a strange notion in our culture that if you've worked really hard, you deserve a big, gooey, sugary treat. Maybe this satisfies emotional longing, but it is certainly not what growing young bodies need for recovery after a game or practice. Using the end of a game as yet another excuse to drink pop, or eat candy, doughnuts and junk food sends the wrong message to the head and the wrong food to the body.

Get clear. What the body needs is some real, wholesome food. What the head and heart need are positive comments about the game that was just played. Remember that the body has been stressed in a good way and nutrients have been used up. Trying to refuel with empty calories like sugary treats does nothing to rebuild what has been lost, and leaves the body yearning for what it's missing. Candy is only sweet for a moment.

The sugary reward system is hard to change. The surest way to shift our culture is for parents and players to receive clear instructions about post-game snacks from coaches. Everyone benefits when players arrive for the next practice or game fit to play.

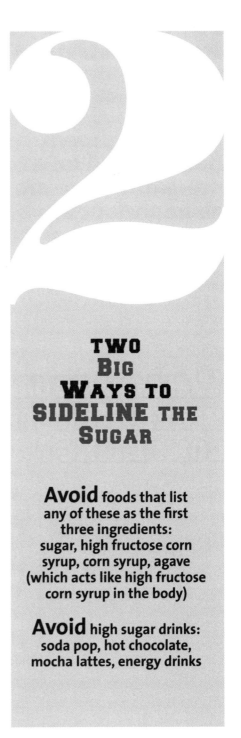

TWO BIG WAYS TO SIDELINE THE SUGAR

Avoid foods that list any of these as the first three ingredients: sugar, high fructose corn syrup, corn syrup, agave (which acts like high fructose corn syrup in the body)

Avoid high sugar drinks: soda pop, hot chocolate, mocha lattes, energy drinks

MAKE YOUR PLATE WHOLE

The right proportions of food on a pre-game plate are as important as what to eat

The pre-game plate gives you a sense of what should take up the biggest amount of space on your plate and what should be kept to a minimum. Percentages are by volume rather than by weight, so it's more of a visual, eyeballing-it guide.

Supercharge by eating grains, chomping fruits and vegetables, putting protein in its place and sidelining the sugar. Fill your plate to look like this:

WHAT ABOUT OFF-SEASON WHEN NOT TRAINING OR COMPETING?

The pre-game plate was designed to prepare you for practice and competition. It is not intended to reflect growing children's and young adults' overall diet. Use the new USDA MyPlate recommendations as a guideline for when there is no game or practice to prime

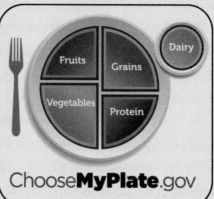

your body for. Note, the protein serving is bigger, grains slightly smaller, and fruits and vegetables cover half the plate—just right for young athletes when not preparing for or recovering from competition.

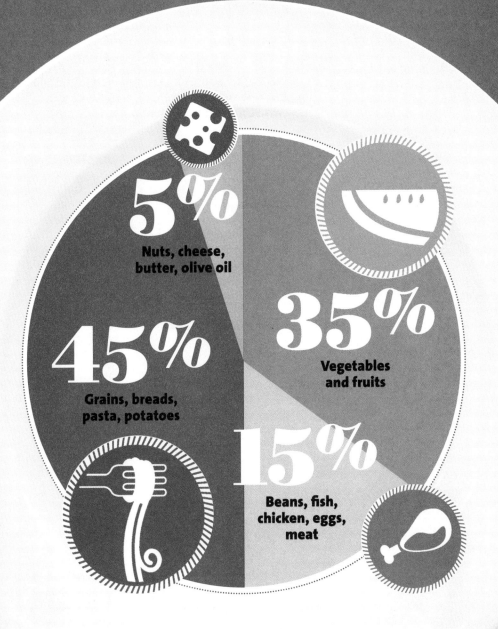

5%
Nuts, cheese,
butter, olive oil

35%
Vegetables
and fruits

45%
Grains, breads,
pasta, potatoes

15%
Beans, fish,
chicken, eggs,
meat

10 WINNING PRE-GAME MEAL IDEAS

GO, TEAM, GO!

1 110% Chicken Noodle Soup served with Whole Grain Bread and Pesto Butter

2 Big Mo Minestrone served with Buttermilk Honey Cornbread

3 Chickpea Broccoli Indian Curry served with Quinoa with Raita Yogurt Topping

4 Mediterranean Lentil, Sweet Potato and Spinach Stew served with Warm Pita and Mint Yogurt

5 Chipotle Black Bean Stew served with Grace's One-Touch Quesadillas

6 Baja Fish Tacos and Lime Slaw served with Creamy Cilantro Sauce

7 Chicken Vegetable Teriyaki served over Brown Rice

8 Edamame Tofu Salad served with Sesame Chili Dressing

9 Samurai Salmon and Avocado Bowl served with Wasabi Dressing

10 Hoppin' John and Chicken Apple Sausage served with Cheesy Polenta

SCORE! CHECK OUT THESE RECIPES on pages 108–123

The post-game snack should be four parts carbohydrates to one part protein

This brings up another key point—the importance of including a small amount of protein in the post-game snack or meal. A 4:1 ratio of carbohydrates to protein stimulates insulin, which helps glucose transform into muscle glycogen. Post-game snack size is important, too. You may feel overwhelmed (even nauseated) looking at a huge plate of food right after playing hard. Picture appetizers. Amuse-bouche. Small bites.

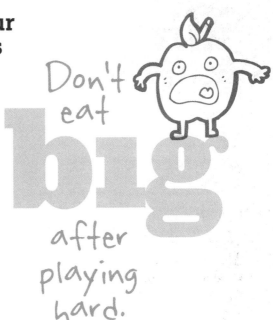

10 QUICK POST-GAME SNACKS

1	2	3	4	5
Whole grain crackers with cheese and grapes	Raisin bread and a banana	Turkey and veggie chapatti roll-ups cut into 2-inch pieces	Half a whole grain bagel with cream cheese	PB & J sandwiches cut into fourths

6	7	8	9	10
Tortilla chips with salsa and bean dip	Fresh vegetables and dip	Rice cakes with almond butter and apples	Homemade oatmeal cookies and oranges	Pita bread and hummus

RELAX, RECOVER, REBUILD

To recover after exercise, players need to drink fluids, eat and relax

The game, the tournament, the challenging practice are over. Now what?

Remember to drink plenty of water and eat a post-game snack right away to take advantage of the glycogen window. Competitive sports can be hard on the body. During exercise your body uses up stored energy in the form of muscle glycogen. The body also produces waste and stress hormones that need to be flushed out. Micro-tears in muscle tissues need to be repaired.

If you don't focus some attention on recovery, your overall progress is slowed down with the potential to become "overtrained," which can end your season early. When you do take time to restore fluids, eat, stretch and rest, you come back stronger the next day.

Put your feet up. Literally.
Once at an out-of-town tournament, with back-to-back games, the players on my daughter's team lay down in a row on the floor of the hotel room, with pillows under head, water bottles in hand, and legs resting straight up against the wall. This restorative yoga pose can work wonders on tired legs. Resting on a bed or on a sofa with your feet on an ottoman will also allow your legs to recover. The backseat of the car works, too.

Eat again if the timing is right.
Take the time to eat if you are hungry. But if it is late at night, and you've had a post-game snack, it's okay to just hit the sack and look forward to a big breakfast in the morning.

Keep sip, sip, sipping.
Keep a water bottle nearby and drink it slowly. Add Lime Boost (page 71) to your water or try the Homemade Sports Drink (page 70) for a refreshing new taste.

Ice strains or sprains.
The sooner the ice is put on the injured area, the more efficiently it works. The process of icing accelerates the healing process by bringing fresh blood to the area, which helps carry off injured cells and replaces them with new cells.

Sleep. Organize your life to get eight to ten hours of sleep every night. If there doesn't seem to be enough time for school, homework, sports and other activities, cut back on something. Without sleep, you can't be successful at school or sports.

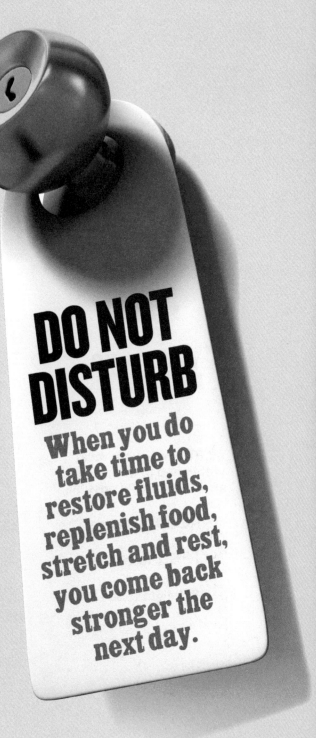

DO NOT DISTURB When you do take time to restore fluids, replenish food, stretch and rest, you come back stronger the next day.

4

FOUR BIG WAYS TO RECOVER

Eat a nutritious meal within two to three hours after the game, if possible

Keep hydrating

Tend to injuries

Sleep eight to ten hours

❗⚫ Don't ignore the demands of travel

My daughter's college soccer team often traveled far for games, which meant long bus rides. Players were told there would be food provided. Unfortunately, a few times there was simply not enough food for 20+ hungry college athletes. My daughter has quick metabolism and gets irritable when her blood sugar drops. She needs food to play well, and she knows it. By mid-season she wised up and started packing some fried rice, a sandwich and a piece of fruit for every trip. She was often asked to share.

Travel zaps energy. Sitting on a plane or a bus for hours sets the body processes, including digestion, on low speed. Dehydration also occurs. Teams that hop on a bus with no plans for how to fuel and hydrate can get caught short-handed. A last-minute trip to a convenience store may be the only food players get.

Plan ahead for trips. Good food and plenty of water in the sports bag are as important as any piece of equipment needed to play.

See ideas for Food on the Road in Chapter 9 (page 125).

GET THE WHOLE TEAM INVOLVED

Everyone benefits when the whole team eats better

Breaking bread together builds community. One of the wonderful things about playing team sports is to be part of a group sharing the same mission. You can extend the team camaraderie to include gatherings around food.

Team meals not only unite players, they are the most entertaining way to emphasize good sports nutrition habits.

We used to have a big team breakfast before the long car ride to out-of-town games. Not only did this ensure that everyone was well fed, the team entered the event with a sense of support and camaraderie. Team meals can also be organized for the night before a big game. See team meal ideas (page 131).

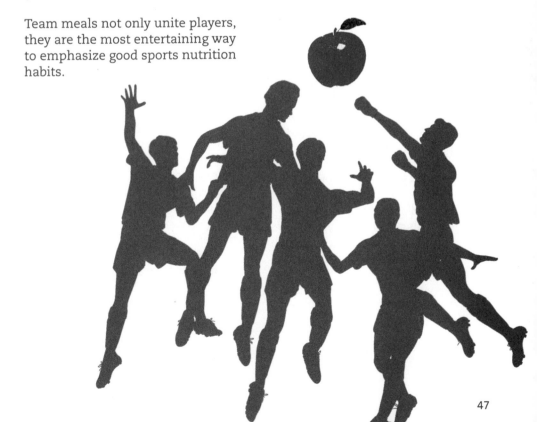

When all players on a team eat to play their best, concentration and endurance during games soar

If each player is dedicated to utilizing good sports nutrition, it adds to team morale. Having common rituals and goals brings the team together, making it a "whole" rather than a group of individuals. Not only will the team's play improve, each player can learn something valuable about the connection between how we eat and how our bodies work.

It may be too hard to imagine how the food you eat today will affect your health when you're in your fifties, but you can see the immediate impact a good morning breakfast has on an afternoon game. If you have a genuine desire to improve your athletic performance, eat better to play your best!

Be a good role model for your teammates and share your knowledge of what, when and how much to eat for optimal performance.

How to get the whole team on board

Team meeting discussion:
Set aside time at a player/parent meeting to talk about feeding young athletes to play their best. Some teams may even dedicate a whole meeting to the subject, followed by a social event with a potluck of post-game foods and snacks to share. Make the talk on sports nutrition fun, engaging and delicious.

Creating a snack list: Along with assigning families to bring snacks to different games, the snack organizer can create a list of great snack ideas with a few notes on which foods and drinks to avoid serving to tired athletes.

Coach's direction: Coaches can direct players to stay hydrated before, during and after games. They can also remind players to eat a good meal before practices or games. Coaches can point out that good sports nutrition will improve the players' health, their games, their concentration, and likely prevent injuries.

Team captain's role: Captains can encourage players to be hydrated and fueled up before, during and after games.

REMEMBER THESE
10 ESSENTIAL GUIDELINES
FOR IMPROVING AND SUSTAINING ATHLETIC PERFORMANCE

Wise up to how foods create energy

Eat using the timetable

Sip, sip, sip

Supercharge with whole grains

Chomp fruits and vegetables

Put protein in its place

Sideline the sugar

Make your plate whole

Relax, recover, rebuild

Get the whole team involved

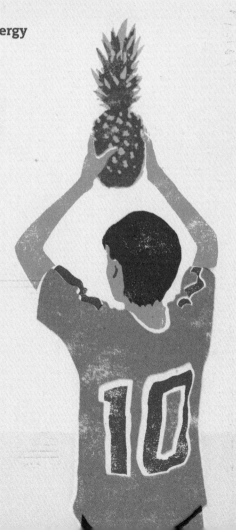

Five Eating Habits That Undermine Performance

Over the years I have observed five common eating habits that undermine performance. They weaken your ability to play your best, and lead to disappointment. You may feel like you've let the team down. If you do, forgive yourself right away. Juggling meals and schedules can be challenging, but the first step is to recognize the problems. Remember that some food is better than no food. Rebalance by eating better soon, and your play will improve immediately. Moving forward, avoid these five bad eating habits.

Don't Do This

Drinking only when thirsty

Skipping meals

Eating on the run

Choosing foods that steal energy

Depending on supplements

DRINKING ONLY WHEN THIRSTY

Sip, sip, sip, even if you're not thirsty

When the body is not well hydrated, extra energy is diverted to regulate body temperature instead of fueling muscles. The body will also steal water from both the bloodstream and from inside the cells in order to cool down, further diminishing muscle function. If this goes on, you can suffer symptoms of heat exhaustion (dizziness, nausea, profuse sweating); heatstroke (hot, dry skin, headaches, rapid pulse, faintness, flushing); and muscle cramps.

By the time you feel thirsty, dehydration has already begun.

Since players may not always feel thirsty in the heat of a game or practice, parents and coaches need to monitor the team's water intake, especially during events held in hot weather. The second most common sports injury among young athletes, and the most preventable, is heat exhaustion or heatstroke.

SKIPPING MEALS

Avoid the two-week slump

At the beginning of the season, your energy and performance levels may seem okay. But experience shows that after two weeks of intense training, players may experience a decline in performance. This "two-week slump" is particularly noticeable for players who have been eating a low carbohydrate diet or skipping meals.

When you are in training or competing weekly, regular meals and snacks keep your motor humming. If you skip meals, you simply do not have the muscle glycogen to keep muscles firing, and your energy will wane dramatically in the second half of games.

Continually skipping meals leads to a slump in overall performance. If you are a regular starter, you may find yourself on the bench. When you keep up a high intake of healthy carbohydrate foods and follow pre-game and post-game eating schedules, your performance level will remain stable game after game.

EATING ON THE RUN

Digestion actually improves in the company of others when the pace of the eating is more leisurely.

Take time to taste your food

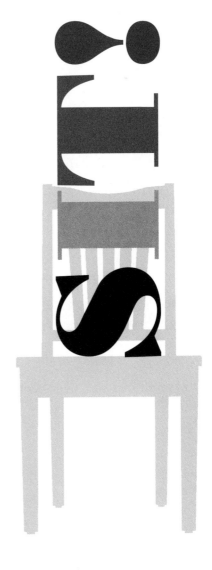

People often stuff food in their mouths on their way out the door, while in the car, or hurrying onto the field. Unfocused eating leads to poor digestion. Athletic performance is jeopardized from lack of fully metabolized food. You may feel gas, bloating, nausea or cramps—not how you want to feel in a game!

When your taste buds give you messages of pleasure, the digestive enzymes in your mouth and stomach come alive and work to break down the food. Sit down to eat.

Do your best not to do anything else while eating. Think of eating as part of your training.

You wouldn't watch TV in the middle of practice. So why do that during dinner? Better to concentrate and taste your food.

CHOOSING FOODS THAT STEAL ENERGY

Skip high-fat, high-sugar foods and caffeine on game days

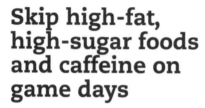 My daughter's U-12 soccer team played all the way to the finals of the Kent Cornucopia Cup tournament. The July weather was hot, and it was the second game of the day, fifth game of the weekend. After the morning semi-final game, we had a break before the hot afternoon championship game.

The opposing Bumble Bees were very nimble and speedy players and had beaten their previous opponents by a wide margin.

We took our team to a shady spot and gave them pasta salads, fruit and plenty of water. Another parent had stayed at the tournament venue and noticed that the Bumble Bees had dined on corn dogs and fries right before game time. The game went pretty much like you might expect. The first half hour the two teams were fairly well matched. Then, the Bumble Bees stopped buzzing. Their energy went to digesting all of the fatty, greasy food in their bellies. They ended up losing by a couple of goals.

Foods high in fat will not leave the stomach, nor will they metabolize quickly enough to give you energy. Foods and beverages that contain sugar and caffeine will give you an initial rush of energy followed by sluggishness or irritability—not good qualities for competitions or practice.

6 FOODS TO AVOID BEFORE A GAME OR EVENT

1	2	3
Cheeseburgers and hamburgers	**Doughnuts and pastries**	**French fries**
4	5	6
Fried chicken or fried fish sandwiches	**Milk shakes and ice cream**	**Pepperoni pizza with double cheese**

DEPENDING ON SUPPLEMENTS

Get your supplements from whole foods

 Why not just take a multivitamin and call it good? Because pills are not the same as food. Look at a pill. It never grew somewhere and it will never die. It is not alive. We eat to bring in the life force of food. We have yet to duplicate that life force in a pill. Remember that they are rightly named a "supplement"— meaning they can't replace food, but can only be an add-on.

Supplements come in a variety of forms.

Remember, supplements can be added to drinks, smoothies, bars, shots, powders and even candy. And, they come with all sorts of promises. Be wary. Read labels.

If you decide to take a supplement, a word of advice from a young athlete I know: "Don't play after you take a supplement without eating food first." So true. Very likely to cause nausea.

PART TWO

WHAT TO FEED YOUNG ATHLETES

Plan ahead.
Choose whole foods.
Strive for balance.

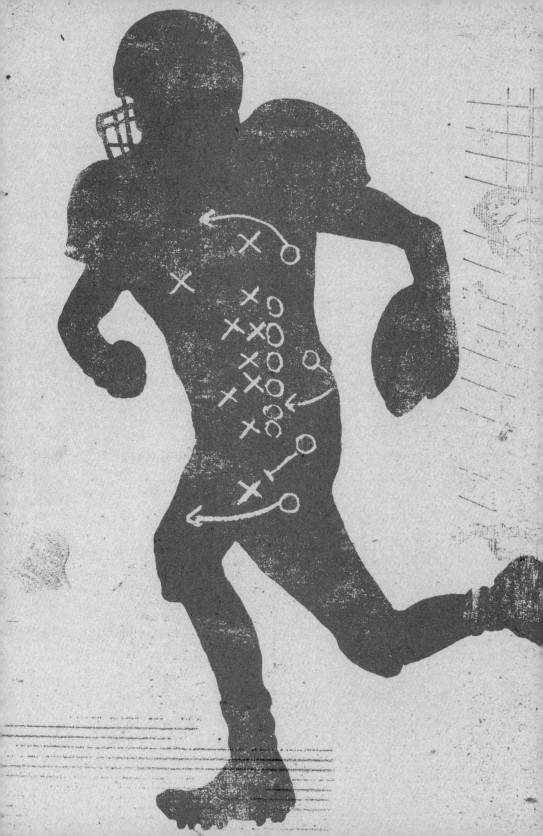

3

Top Ten Foods for Your Game Plan

Eat This

Whole grains: Quinoa

Fruits: Blueberries

Dark greens: Spinach

Orange vegetables: Sweet potatoes

Legumes: Lentils

Vegetarian protein: Free-range eggs

Animal protein: Wild-caught salmon

Dairy: Yogurt

Nuts & seeds: Almonds

Cooking fats: Olive oil

Mother Nature provides a bounty of nutrient-dense whole foods that help you grow, move and flourish

There are so many good foods! Eating better to play your best can be delicious and nourishing. In choosing the foods listed in this chapter, we asked ourselves:

Is it a whole food?
Is it nutrient rich?
Is it widely available?
Is it versatile in recipes?

WHOLE GRAINS

Though it is technically a seed, **quinoa** [KEEN-wah] is known as the "mother grain" to the Incas of South America. Quinoa contains essential amino acids and has a higher protein profile than most whole grains. Quinoa also contains calcium and iron. Even better, it cooks in 15 minutes and has a lovely nutty flavor. Red and black quinoa adds beautiful color to any dish while providing vital carbohydrates for building muscle glycogen.

Other winners: steel-cut oats, brown rice

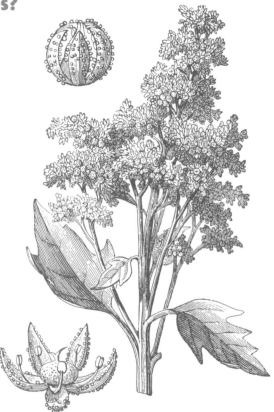

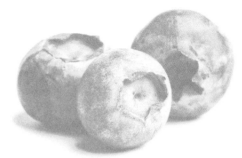

FRUITS

Blueberries are bite-sized pops of sweet nourishment that are native to the North American landscape. They have high levels of phytonutrients, which are non-vitamin, non-mineral components of food that help our cells communicate with each other more efficiently— a definite plus when you need to create energy quickly.

Other winners: watermelon, apples

ORANGE VEGETABLES

Orange-fleshed **sweet potatoes** are one of nature's unsurpassed sources of beta-carotene. Good for

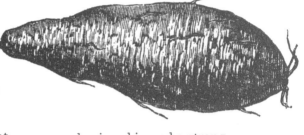

eyes, glowing skin and a strong immune system, beta-carotene is enhanced in the presence of small amounts of fat. So put some butter on your baked sweet potatoes or roast them in olive oil. Yum!

Other winners: carrots, winter squash

DARK GREENS

Spinach is nutrient-dense, readily available in grocery stores, and a tasty addition to egg dishes, soups and salads. It is full of vitamins, minerals and health-promoting phytonutrients such as carotenoids and flavonoids. Plus, it cooks in seconds. Spinach and other dark leafy greens are rich in bioavailable calcium to help support bone growth.

Other winners: kale, broccoli

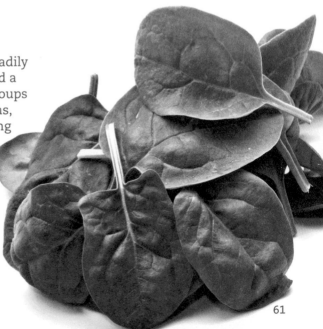

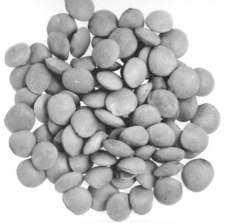

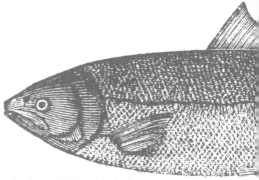

LEGUMES

Lentils are loaded with protein, fiber and iron. They are the Environmental Working Group's top choice for a climate-friendly protein and an excellent vegan protein. Combine lentils and vegetables and serve them with whole grains for a hearty pre-game meal. Ladle up some soup!

Other winners: black beans, chickpeas

ANIMAL PROTEIN

Wild-caught salmon is expensive, but you don't need a huge portion to reap its benefits. Remember, four to six ounces of protein a day is all that our bodies can absorb. Salmon is renowned for its abundant omega-3 fatty acids, which keep inflammation in check. Serve high-quality protein foods as a side dish or flavoring in the pre-game meal.

Other winners: grass-fed beef, free-range chicken

VEGETARIAN PROTEIN

The amino acids in **free-range eggs** are perfectly aligned to meet your protein needs. If the eggs are from pasture-raised chickens, they will be rich in vitamins A, D and E, beta-carotene, and omega-3 fatty acids. Whoa! These nutrients help fight inflammation, support good eyesight and promote bone growth. Enjoy eggs and stay fit to play.

Other winners (vegan): tofu, miso

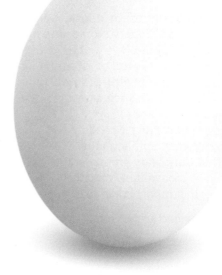

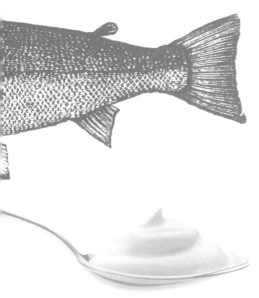

NUTS AND SEEDS

A quarter cup of **almonds** contains healthy fats, vitamin E, potassium and almost 99 mg of magnesium. When there is enough magnesium around, veins and arteries breathe a sigh of relief and relax, improving the flow of blood, oxygen and nutrients throughout the body. Potassium is an important electrolyte involved in nerve transmission and muscle contraction. These qualities make almonds a superior snack for athletes.

Other winners: walnuts, sunflower seeds

DAIRY

Yogurt is made by inoculating milk with friendly bacteria (or probiotics). This process results in a creamy and easy-to-digest food that is delicious with cereals, fruits and nuts. The friendly bacteria also keep the immune system strong. For athletes, this means readily available protein and carbohydrates, plus the protection of probiotics. Be sure to look for yogurt that does not contain a lot of sugar, artificial sweeteners or coloring.

Other winners: mozzarella, milk

COOKING FATS

Olive oil is very versatile as it can be used for salad dressings as well as cooking vegetables. Not only does olive oil have anti-inflammatory properties, it is a very stable fat—meaning it does not spoil easily. While all oils are "un-whole" (e.g., the oil is removed from the olive), some are more healthful than others.

Other winners: butter, unrefined sesame oil

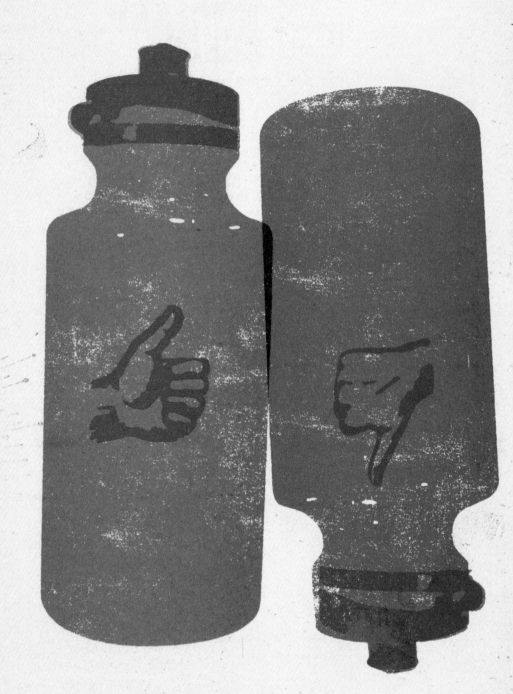

CHAPTER 4

Homemade Sports Drinks

Drink This

Water

Homemade Sports Drink

Fresh Lemonade Hydrator

Lime Boost

Diluted lemonade

Naturally flavored water

Coconut water

Don't Drink This

Carbonated drinks

Artificially sweetened drinks

Caffeinated drinks

Energy drinks

Unfiltered apple juice

Milk as a hydration drink

Water is the best, hands down

Now that you understand how crucial hydration is to playing your best game, the logical question is, "What should I drink?" Plain old water is a great choice, especially if you're already eating fruit and other carbohydrate-containing foods to keep up your energy.

The American Academy of Pediatrics recommends that children and adolescents drink plain water for "hydration before, during, and after most exercise regimens."

Research on adult athletes demonstrates that, under extreme physical exertion and environmental conditions, the addition of small amounts of carbohydrates, sodium and potassium will enhance the rate of fluid absorption. Recommendations for carbohydrate concentration range from 2% to 8% (5 to 18 grams of simple sugars), with amounts above 8% actually slowing fluid absorption.

Drink cool water, not cold water. Between 59°F and 72°F is just right.

An excellent sports drink can be made at home without the high fructose corn syrup, artificial flavorings, chemicals and colorings that show up in commercial sports beverages. Remember that commercial sports drinks not only add unnecessary ingredients, but also calories and cost.

Try a homemade sports drink for nonstop endurance sports played in hot conditions

A homemade sports drink jazzes up the taste of plain water, motivating you to drink more. This can be effective when playing hockey, football, soccer, basketball and other high-performance sports, especially in hot, humid weather or in a hot, stuffy gym. In these circumstances, you can lose a significant percentage of body weight through perspiration and will need to replace electrolytes and fluids.

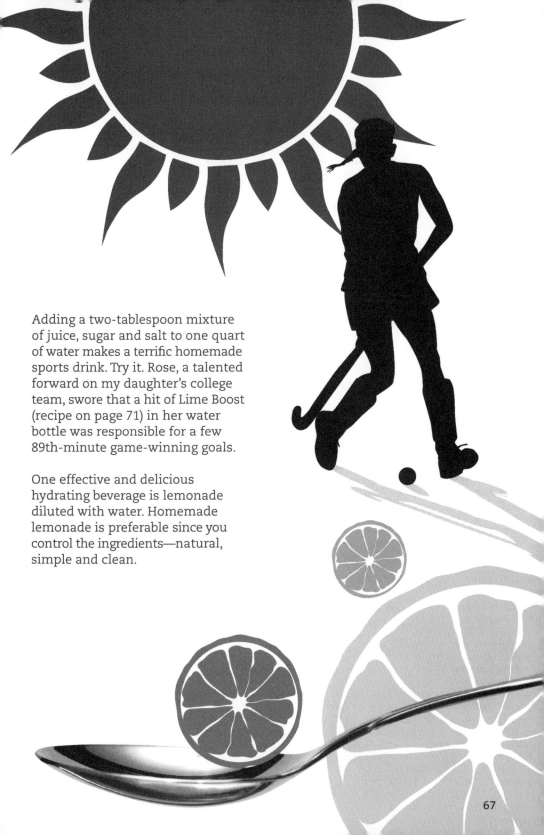

Adding a two-tablespoon mixture of juice, sugar and salt to one quart of water makes a terrific homemade sports drink. Try it. Rose, a talented forward on my daughter's college team, swore that a hit of Lime Boost (recipe on page 71) in her water bottle was responsible for a few 89th-minute game-winning goals.

One effective and delicious hydrating beverage is lemonade diluted with water. Homemade lemonade is preferable since you control the ingredients—natural, simple and clean.

Hydration 101

The news that flavors in water aid hydration has spawned a new breed of commercial "flavored waters." Use caution and read labels. Do not buy flavored waters that contain unrecognizable ingredients, vitamins, herbs, and other additives and supplements. Adding your own natural flavors at home is very easy and much less expensive. If you wish, buy flavored waters that contain water and only a small amount of natural flavoring.

New on the rehydration scene… coconut water. Sales of coconut water have skyrocketed, largely because of its reputation as a healthy and natural source of electrolytes. The carbohydrate concentration of pure coconut water is between 2% and 5%, falling in the appropriate range. It is an acceptable choice if you like the flavor and you're willing to pay extra for it. Since it's unlikely you will be cracking open a coconut yourself, remember to check the ingredient list to make sure additional "stuff" wasn't added.

Carbonated drinks change the pH levels in the stomach and can cause belching and gas—undesirable when playing sports. Carbonation is the process of dissolving carbon dioxide, under high pressure, in water. When the pressure is reduced, carbon dioxide is released from the solution as small bubbles, which causes the solution to "fizz" in your glass and in your stomach. Soda pop should be avoided anyway. Too much sugar, too many additives.

Caffeinated beverages will not help you hydrate. Caffeine causes frequent urination, which contributes to dehydration. It can also irritate the stomach lining and cause nervousness and shaking. Remember that the typical effect caffeine has on adults is intensified in children and adolescents. No lattes or mochas for young athletes, please.

The stimulants in energy drinks are bad for growing players. The term "energy" refers to substances that act as non-nutritive stimulants, not real energy needed by muscles. Energy drinks are often marketed as performance enhancers, but actually cause jitters and unfocused excitement. Avoid these additives in beverages: caffeine, guarana, taurine, ginseng, I-carnitine, creatine and/or glucuronolactone uronolactone.

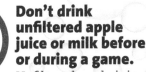 **Don't drink unfiltered apple juice or milk before or during a game.** Unfiltered apple juice and cow's milk can cause stomach cramping in some players. Milk is a high-protein and high-sugar FOOD, not actually a drink if you consider the amount of calories and nutrients it contains. If you choose to drink milk as part of your diet, it's best not to drink it right before or during a game.

Lay off the moo juice before or during a game!

Homemade Sports Drink

Do it yourself and be good to your body. This recipe makes a carbohydrate concentration of 6% that's right in the ideal range. Do not use unfiltered apple juice, as it may cause cramping.

½ cup 100% orange (or other fruit) juice
½ cup sugar
¼ teaspoon sea salt
2 quarts water

▶ Combine juice, sugar and sea salt in pitcher. Stir until salt is dissolved.
▶ Add water and stir more.
▶ Pour into sports bottles.

PREP TIME: 2 minutes
MAKES: over 2 quarts

Fresh Lemonade Hydrator

It's hard to find pre-made lemonade that doesn't contain high fructose corn syrup or other chemical sweeteners. This made-from-scratch drink refreshes hot, tired players all-naturally. Add lemon zest (from the lemon peel) for an extra pop of citrus.

2 cups water
¾ cup fresh lemon juice
½ cup sugar or sucanat
   (dehydrated whole cane sugar)
2 teaspoons lemon zest, minced
1½ quarts additional water

▶ Bring water to boil in saucepan. Add lemon juice, sugar and zest. Reduce to simmer. Stir until sugar dissolves. Let cool.
▶ Pour into pitcher, and add water to bring up to 2 quarts.
▶ Pour into sports bottles.

PREP TIME: 15 minutes
MAKES: 2 quarts

Remember

1 quart = slightly under 1 liter
4 cups = 1 quart

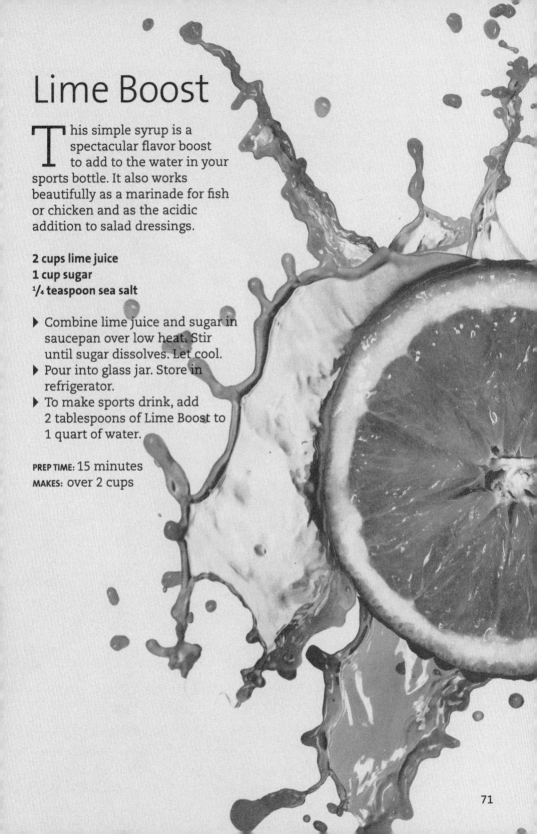

Lime Boost

This simple syrup is a spectacular flavor boost to add to the water in your sports bottle. It also works beautifully as a marinade for fish or chicken and as the acidic addition to salad dressings.

2 cups lime juice
1 cup sugar
¼ teaspoon sea salt

▸ Combine lime juice and sugar in saucepan over low heat. Stir until sugar dissolves. Let cool.
▸ Pour into glass jar. Store in refrigerator.
▸ To make sports drink, add 2 tablespoons of Lime Boost to 1 quart of water.

PREP TIME: 15 minutes
MAKES: over 2 cups

71

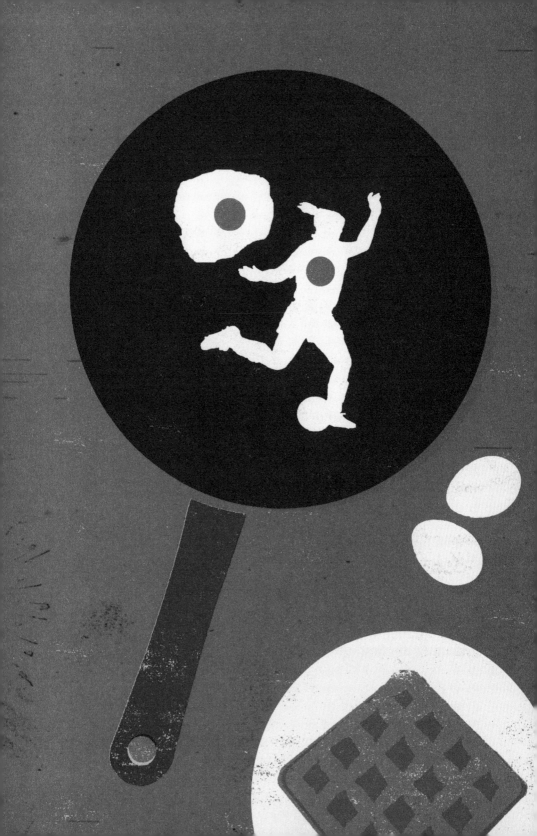

5

Breakaway Breakfast Recipes

Make This

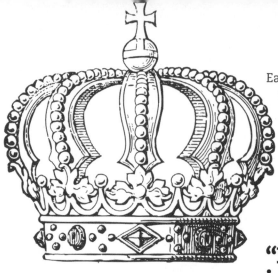

Eating sugary cereal topped with milk or pastries laden with refined sugar will not sustain your body, whether you're gearing up for an athletic event or not. America may be a hotbed of innovation, but you wouldn't know it by looking at its breakfast bowl.

"But I'm not hungry in the morning."

"Eat breakfast like a king" is good advice

Simple solution—don't eat late at night. Stop snacking after dinner so that when you go to bed the body can rest and repair instead of churning to digest food. You'll wake up well-rested and ready to eat your morning meal.

Breakfast sets the metabolic rhythm for the day. Like the farmer preparing for a day of physical labor, the athlete needs to make sure the morning meal has complex carbohydrates, protein, fat and fiber. A breakfast with all four provides you with a steady energy supply to play your best.

It's high time we thought outside the cereal box.

! ● Skip breakfast and you'll hit a slump mid-morning

When you skip breakfast, your thinking goes blurry, your muscles feel droopy, and you may find yourself playing catch-up all day with too many snacks.

Get involved in the meal preparation—planning, shopping, cooking—whenever possible

Setting the table or cutting up apples count. You can also help plan the weekly menu, write out shopping lists, find items at the store, and start learning basic cooking skills. Think of the recipes here as a primer in whole foods cooking, designed specifically for young athletes who want to play their best game. Some of the recipes require time and planning, but several are quick and easy to prepare.

We've included recipes for popular breakfast foods such as pancakes, waffles and oatmeal. A few global recipes are inspired by Chinese, Korean and Mexican ingredients and cooking techniques. Two of the recipes are flavorful twists on home fries. There's a smoothie recipe, of course. And, a bagel and lox that pays homage to my home in the Pacific Northwest, also known as the Salmon Nation.

Videos that show you how to prepare many of the recipes in this book can be found at my online cooking program, *www.cookus.tv*.

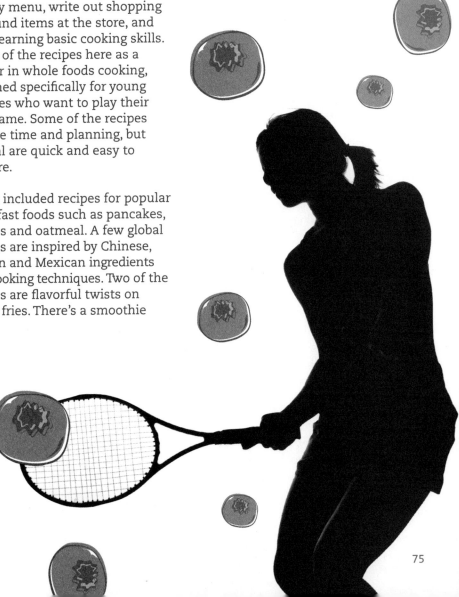

75

Whole Grain Banana Flapjacks

Making your own pancake mix is easier than you may think, and you get to choose which whole grain flours you want. This pancake mix can be doubled or tripled and stored in an airtight container. Adding in stiff egg whites makes for extra-fluffy pancakes. If you need to, substitute buttermilk with one cup milk and one tablespoon vinegar, or with yogurt and enough water to reach the correct consistency.

Dry pancake mix:
½ cup barley or kamut flour
¾ cup whole wheat pastry flour
¼ cup buckwheat flour
1 tablespoon baking powder
½ teaspoon nutmeg
½ teaspoon sea salt

▸ Combine all ingredients.
▸ For a gluten-free pancake mix, skip the barley and whole wheat pastry flour and use the following instead:
1¼ cup rice flour, 2 tablespoons potato starch and 2 tablespoons tapioca flour. The buckwheat flour is gluten-free, so it can stay.

PREP TIME: 5 minutes
MAKES: 1½ cups pancake mix
Vegetarian, Nut-free, Gluten-free option

Flapjacks:
1 egg
1½ cups pancake mix
1 cup buttermilk
½ cup water
1 ripe banana, sliced
Oil for the griddle
Maple syrup and butter to serve

▸ Separate egg whites and yolk into 2 mixing bowls. Beat egg whites with mixer until stiff peaks form. Set aside.
▸ Combine egg yolk, pancake mix, buttermilk and water. Mix well. Gently fold egg whites into batter.
▸ Add oil to hot griddle or skillet. Pour batter onto griddle to form 5-inch-diameter pancakes. Place a few banana slices on top.
▸ When tiny bubbles form, flip and cook other side.
▸ Serve with butter and maple syrup.

PREP TIME: 30 minutes
MAKES: 10 pancakes
Vegetarian, Nut-free, Gluten-free option

Overnight Oat Waffles

Prepare breakfast overnight ... while you're dreaming! Soaking grains makes them more digestible. Use vanilla yogurt if you want sweeter waffles. Start the sauce once you get the waffles going. A potato masher works well to smoosh sauce.

Waffles:
2 cups rolled oats
½ cup plain whole milk yogurt
¾ cup water
1 egg
¼ teaspoon sea salt
2 tablespoons brown sugar or sucanat
 (dehydrated whole cane sugar)
1 teaspoon baking powder
½ teaspoon grated nutmeg

▶ Combine oats, yogurt and water in blender. Cover and soak overnight in refrigerator.
▶ In the morning, preheat waffle iron.
▶ Blend oats mixture with remaining ingredients in blender until smooth.
▶ Pour about ¼ cup batter onto hot oiled griddle. Close and cook for about 2 minutes or until golden.
▶ Serve with butter and warm strawberry rhubarb sauce.

PREP TIME: 30 minutes (plus overnight soaking)
MAKES: 4 waffles
Vegetarian, Nut-free, Gluten-free

Strawberry rhubarb sauce:
2 tablespoons brown sugar or sucanat
 (dehydrated whole cane sugar)
2 tablespoons water
¼ cup rhubarb, diced
1 cup strawberries, hulled and halved
1 teaspoon lemon juice

▶ Combine sugar and water in saucepan over medium heat. Stir until sugar dissolves.
▶ Add rhubarb. Reduce to simmer, cover and cook 15 minutes, or until tender.
▶ Add strawberries and lemon juice. Simmer 10 minutes more.
▶ Use your potato masher or wooden spoon to press down cooked fruit until it looks like a thick sauce.

PREP TIME: 15 minutes
MAKES: ¾ cup sauce
Vegetarian, Nut-free, Gluten-free

Steel-Cut Oats with Almond Butter and Blueberries

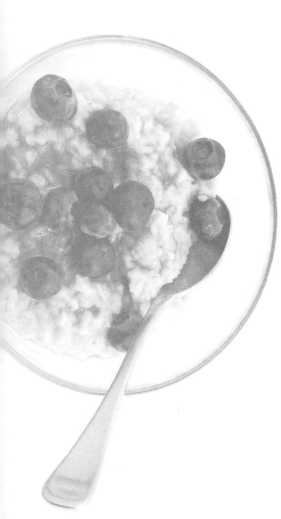

Steel-cut oats are whole oats that have been cut into pieces. They are different from rolled oats, which have been heated until soft, then pressed flat. Steel-cut oats, sometimes called Irish oatmeal, have a nuttier flavor and a chewier texture than rolled oats.

1 cup steel-cut oats
3 cups water
½ teaspoon sea salt
1 tablespoon almond butter
1 cup blueberries

▸ Soak oats overnight in 2-quart pan with 3 cups water.
▸ In the morning, add salt. Bring to boil, reduce to simmer, and stir constantly for 5 minutes, or until mixture is creamy.
▸ Stir in almond butter.
▸ If you're using frozen blueberries, stir them into hot cereal and cook until warm. You can add fresh blueberries right on top of the cereal in the bowl.

PREP TIME: 10 minutes
(plus overnight soaking)
MAKES: 4 to 6 servings
Vegetarian, Gluten-free

Chinese Vegetable Fried Rice

Open your mind. Breakfast doesn't have to be sweet. How about a savory start to the day? Rice is the principal food for half the world's people. With cooked brown rice on hand, prep time is only a few minutes. For fluffier rice, no peeking or stirring while it cooks! This dish works well as a one-bowl lunch or dinner too.

Brown rice:
1½ cup brown rice
2½ cups water
Pinch of sea salt

▶ Rinse and drain rice.
▶ Combine rice, water and salt in pot. Bring to low boil, reduce to simmer, and cover. Cook 45 minutes, or until all water is absorbed.

PREP TIME: 50 minutes
MAKES: 4 cups
Vegetarian, Nut-free, Gluten-free

Fried rice:
3 eggs
1 carrot, diced
½ cup peas
6 teaspoons coconut or other high-heat vegetable oil
1 teaspoon toasted sesame oil
4 cups cooked brown rice
Salt and pepper to taste
2 tablespoons tamari (naturally brewed soy sauce)
2 scallions, sliced
Hot pepper sesame oil, optional

▶ Whisk eggs in bowl. Add 2 teaspoons vegetable oil to hot wok (or skillet). Add eggs. Fold over eggs by lifting from bottom until softly cooked. Set aside.
▶ Add 2 more teaspoons vegetable oil to hot wok. Add carrots and peas. Stir-fry until tender. Set aside.
▶ Add remaining vegetable oil, sesame oil and cooked brown rice to wok. Stir-fry constantly. If you like a crispy edge, let rice cook for 1-2 minutes before flipping over.
▶ Add back in cooked eggs, carrots and peas. Salt and pepper to taste. Stir-fry to mix ingredients together.
▶ Add tamari and scallions. Stir-fry again to mix flavors.
▶ Divide into bowls. Dragon types who like fire can top rice with several drops of hot pepper oil.

PREP TIME: 15 minutes
MAKES: 4 servings
Vegetarian, Nut-free, Gluten-free

Be Bop Breakfast

This is a spin-off on the traditional Korean rice dish, Bibimbap. I like to cook it in my large cast-iron skillet for quick and even heating. Serve with fermented cabbage, either kimchi or sauerkraut, to add more flavor and a dose of friendly bacteria (or probiotics). Be Bop is the breakfast of champions, so have a super-charged morning!

6 teaspoons butter
2 scallions, chopped
2 cups cooked brown rice
4 kale leaves, cut into ribbons
2 eggs
Tamari (naturally brewed soy sauce) to taste
Apple cider vinegar to taste
Kimchi or sauerkraut, optional
Thai chili sauce, optional

▸ Add 2 teaspoons butter and scallions to hot skillet. When scallions are bright green, add cooked rice. Stir-fry until thoroughly heated. Divide rice into 2 large bowls. Drizzle tamari to taste. Set aside.

▸ Add 2 teaspoons of butter and kale to hot skillet until kale is just wilted and glistening. Add 2 tablespoons of water and cover until kale is tender.

▸ Divide kale on top of rice bowls. Sprinkle vinegar to taste. Set aside.

▸ Add remaining butter to skillet, and heat until sizzling. Break eggs into skillet and cook sunny-side-up or over easy.

▸ Top each bowl with 1 fried egg.

▸ Trail some tamari and Thai chili sauce on top if you like heat. Garnish with kimchi or sauerkraut.

PREP TIME: 15 minutes
MAKES: 2 servings
Vegetarian, Nut-free, Gluten-free

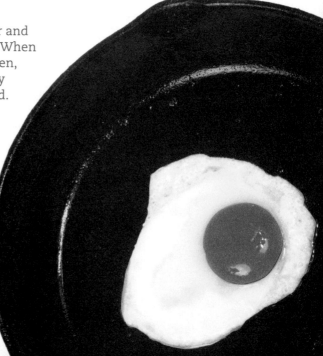

Green Eggs (No Ham!) Breakfast Burrito

Breakfast burritos are warm, satisfying, and quick to make. The water clinging to the washed spinach provides enough moisture for cooking. Taste the cheese you plan to use before cooking the eggs. If it's salty, use less salt on the eggs.

1 cup baby spinach leaves
4 whole wheat tortillas
5 eggs
1 tablespoon water or milk
1½ tablespoons butter
Salt to taste
¼ cup grated cheese, your choice
Salsa or fresh pico de gallo (page 98)

▸ Cook spinach on hot skillet until wilted. Drain, chop and set aside.
▸ Place tortillas in covered pan in warm oven.
▸ Whisk eggs and water (or milk) in bowl. Add butter to hot skillet. Add egg mixture. Fold over eggs by lifting from bottom until nearly cooked. Turn off heat.
▸ Add spinach, cheese and salt to taste. Fold to incorporate spinach and cheese.
▸ Place green eggs down the middle of each tortilla. Wrap two sides over eggs, and tuck in ends to make the burrito.
▸ Serve warm with salsa or pico de gallo. (page 98)

PREP TIME: 15 minutes
MAKES: 4 servings
Vegetarian, Nut-free

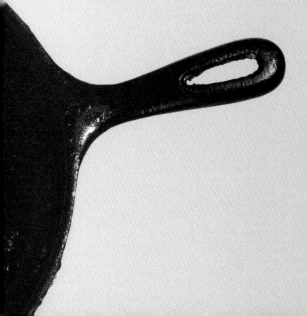

Roasted Garlic Potatoes with Poached Eggs

I like to keep roasted vegetables around to make quick meals, hearty breakfasts and just plain delectable snacks. If you already have some Roasted Garlic Potatoes handy, all you have to do is heat them up in a skillet and make poached eggs.

Roasted potatoes:
12 small red potatoes, halved or quartered
5 cloves garlic, minced
1 teaspoon sea salt
3 tablespoons extra-virgin olive oil
Pepper to taste

▸ Preheat oven to 375°F.
▸ Put halved potatoes in large baking pan. Combine minced garlic, salt and olive oil in small bowl. Drizzle over potatoes. Shake pan to coat.
▸ Roast 45 minutes, or until potatoes are tender inside and browned outside.
▸ Divide up roasted potatoes onto 4 plates. Store extra in refrigerator.

Poached eggs:
4 eggs
½ teaspoon vinegar
Salt and pepper to taste

▸ Bring 2-quart pot of water to low boil. Add vinegar.
▸ Break open an egg in small bowl.
▸ Stir water clockwise until a vortex forms in the middle. Gently drop egg in center of vortex.
▸ Set timer for 3 minutes for a runny yolk, 4 minutes for a slightly set yolk.
▸ Remove poached egg with slotted spoon. Repeat with other eggs.
▸ Serve with roasted potatoes. Salt and pepper to taste.

PREP TIME: 50 minutes
MAKES: 4 servings
Vegetarian, Nut-free, Gluten-free

Roasted Sweet Potatoes with Cinnamon

Eating nutrient-rich sweet potatoes for breakfast satisfies your morning sweet craving while providing sustained energy to get you through the day. You can prep the vegetable and fruit the night before, so the oven can do all the work for you in the morning. Dicing up the potatoes into one-inch bite sizes reduces bake time and increases deliciousness. Serve without yogurt for a vegan option.

3-4 sweet potatoes, diced into 1-inch pieces
1 apple, diced
3 tablespoons extra-virgin olive oil
1½ teaspoons cinnamon
½ teaspoon salt
¼ cup vanilla yogurt to serve

▶ Preheat oven to 375°F.
▶ Put diced sweet potatoes and apples in 9x13-inch baking pan. Combine olive oil, cinnamon and salt in small bowl. Drizzle over sweet potato mix.
▶ Roast 30 minutes, or until sweet potato chunks split easily with side of a fork.
▶ Serve with yogurt for added protein.

PREP TIME: 40 minutes
MAKES: 4 servings
Vegetarian, Nut-free, Gluten-free

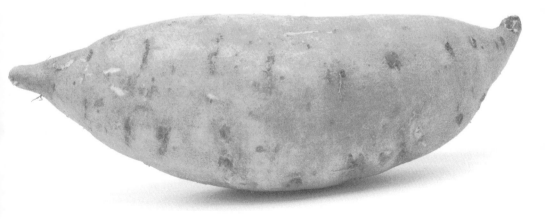

Psyched-Up Smoothie and Raisin Bread Sandwich

Share the smoothie and sandwich with a parent or sibling to have just enough (and not too much) for game day. Substitute whole wheat bread with a gluten-free option if needed.

Smoothie:
1 ripe banana
1 cup frozen fruit
1 cup fruit juice
½ cup yogurt
2 teaspoons sweetener
   (honey, maple syrup or sugar)

▸ Blend banana, fruit, juice, yogurt and sweetener in blender until smooth.

Sandwich:
2 slices whole grain raisin bread
1 teaspoon butter
2 tablespoons almond or peanut butter

▸ Toast bread. Spread on butter and nut butter. Cut in half.
▸ Serve half sandwich with half of the smoothie.

PREP TIME: 5 minutes
MAKES: 2 servings
Vegetarian, Gluten-free option

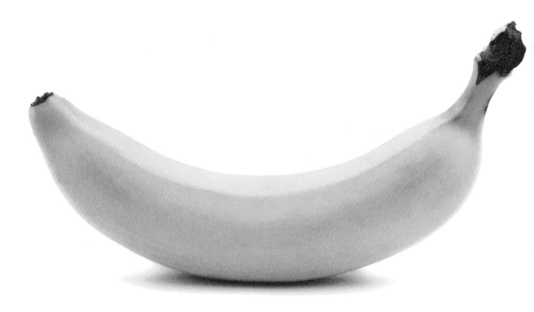

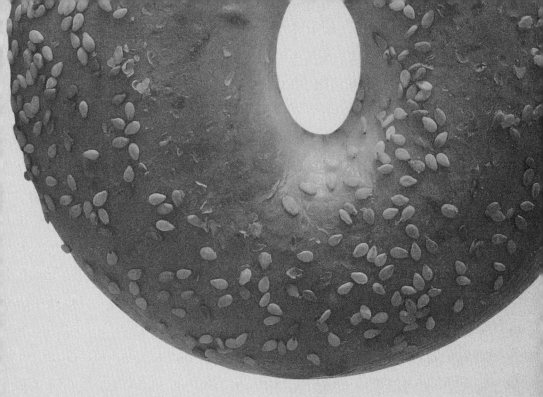

Salmon and Bagels

This simple, satisfying and savory breakfast is a personal favorite of mine. No sugar highs. Just steady energy all morning and an omega-3 boost for the day. Artfully arrange salmon, cut vegetables, capers and spreads on a platter for a make-it-your-own breakfast buffet. But no matter how busy you are, always remember to chew slowly as you enjoy.

2 whole grain bagels
2 teaspoons butter
4 tablespoons cream cheese
2 ounces lox (thinly sliced, cured salmon) or smoked salmon
Capers
Sliced red onion
Sliced tomato

▶ Bisect bagels. Toast and butter each half.
▶ Spread 1 tablespoon cream cheese on each half. Top with 2 or 3 pieces of lox, capers, red onions and tomato.

PREP TIME: 10 minutes
MAKES: 2 big or 4 small servings
Nut-free

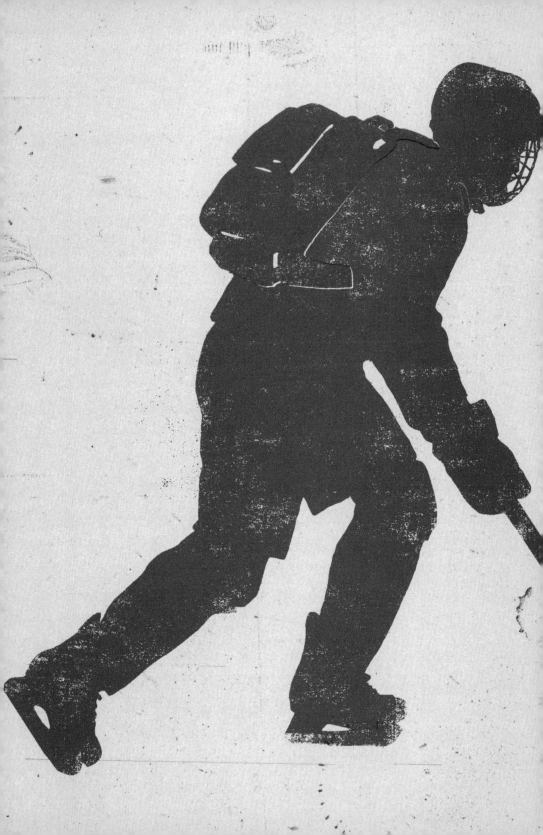

6

Pack-n-Go Snacks to Make in Your Kitchen

Make This

Buttermilk Honey Cornbread

Blast-Off Banana Date Bread

Coconut Date Bonbons and Oranges

Gingerbread Molasses Cookies and Pears

Best Spice-Kissed Oatmeal Raisin Cookies

Peanut Butter Cranberry Zoom Zoom Bars

Tamari Roasted Nuts and Dried Apricots

Rice Cakes with Almond Butter and Melon Mélange

Tortilla Chips and Summery Pico de Gallo

Lemony Hummus with Crispy Vegetables

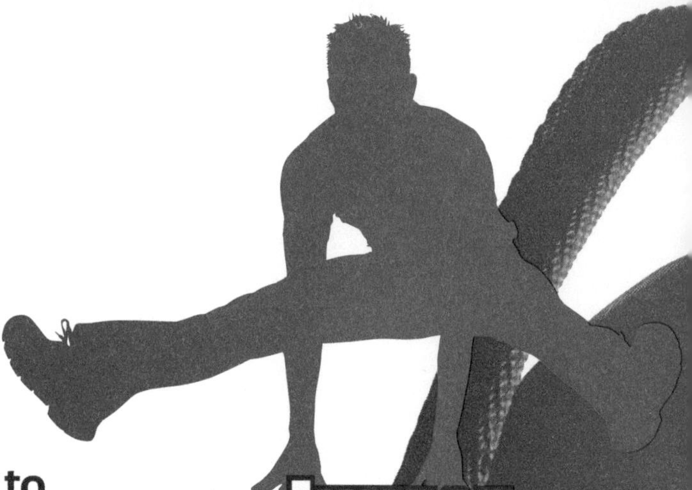

Plan ahead to play your best

We can't stress enough how important it is to plan meals and snacks so that you are fueled and ready to play . . . whether it's the first game of the week or the fourth event of the day. Enlist parents to shop or cook on off-days so that your food is ready to grab-and-go when you need it.

Always have these items in your sports bag:

2 liters of water
1-2 sandwiches
1-2 pieces of fruit

INVEST IN SOME REUSABLE GEAR SO THAT FOOD CAN BE READY TO GO

WE RECOMMEND

1. A soft zippered, insulated, water-resistant lunch box. Always have this filled with food and ready to throw in your athletic bag.

2. Reusable ice packs. Having two or three means there's always one in the freezer for the next game.

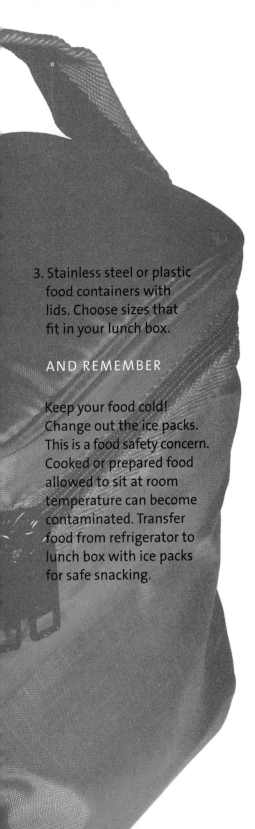

3. Stainless steel or plastic food containers with lids. Choose sizes that fit in your lunch box.

AND REMEMBER

Keep your food cold! Change out the ice packs. This is a food safety concern. Cooked or prepared food allowed to sit at room temperature can become contaminated. Transfer food from refrigerator to lunch box with ice packs for safe snacking.

The more involved you are with your food preparation, the more you'll enjoy eating it

Getting involved with food teaches you valuable life skills, such as planning ahead, contributing to the needs of others and of course, the most basic life skill—feeding yourself whole foods.

Baking and making snacks are fun bonding activities for families and teams.

Unlike cooking, which is an everyday necessity, baking can be planned for days when everyone has more time and energy. The payoff is your happy, satisfied friends and family. So try making these snacks together with your family and teammates. It's easy to double and triple the recipes so you'll have enough to share and some to pack for later.

Videos that demonstrate how to prepare many of the recipes in this book can be found at my online cooking program, *www.cookus.tv*.

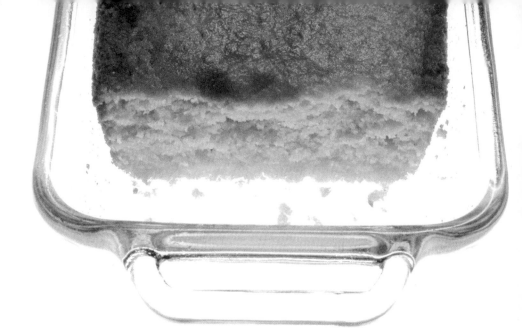

Buttermilk Honey Cornbread

I s there anything more satisfying than cornbread? Carry a slice in your sports bag to take advantage of the post-game glycogen window. Enjoy warm with hot soup, like Big Mo Minestrone (page 110), as a pre-game meal or snack. If you need to, substitute buttermilk with one cup milk and one tablespoon vinegar, or with yogurt and enough water to reach the correct consistency.

1 cup unbleached white flour
1 cup fine cornmeal
1½ teaspoons baking powder
½ teaspoon baking soda
½ teaspoon sea salt
2 eggs
¼ cup honey
¼ cup buttermilk
4 tablespoons butter, melted
¾ cup corn kernels, fresh or frozen

▸ Preheat oven to 350°F.
▸ Mix flour, cornmeal, baking powder, baking soda and sea salt in large bowl. Set aside.
▸ In small bowl, beat eggs. Add honey, buttermilk and melted butter.
▸ Fold wet mixture into dry ingredients. Fold in corn kernels.
▸ Pour batter into lightly greased loaf pan or cupcake tin.
▸ Bake 30 minutes, or until golden brown and springy to touch.

PREP TIME: 40 minutes
MAKES: 1 loaf or 8 thick slices
Vegetarian, Nut-free

Blast-Off Banana Date Bread

This moist and luscious bread relies on bananas, orange juice, dried dates and raisins for natural sweetness. To get extra sweetness from bananas, peel overripe ones and freeze. Thaw before using. It's a great post-practice snack to pack in the sports bag.

1 cup whole wheat pastry flour
1 cup unbleached white flour
2 teaspoons baking powder
1 teaspoon baking soda
½ teaspoon sea salt
2 ripe bananas
¼ cup unsalted butter, melted
10 pitted dates, chopped in pieces
½ cup orange juice
½ cup maple syrup
1 teaspoon vanilla
1 egg
¼ cup walnuts, chopped
½ cup raisins or currants

▶ Preheat oven to 375°F.
▶ Mix flours, baking powder, baking soda and sea salt in large bowl. Set aside.
▶ Blend bananas, butter, dates, juice, maple syrup and vanilla in blender until smooth. Add egg and pulse briefly.
▶ Fold wet mixture into dry ingredients. Fold in nuts and raisins.
▶ Put batter in lightly oiled 8x8-inch baking dish.
▶ Bake 40 minutes, or until knife inserted in center comes out clean.

PREP TIME: 50 minutes
MAKES: 9 to 12 squares, depending on number of cuts
Vegetarian

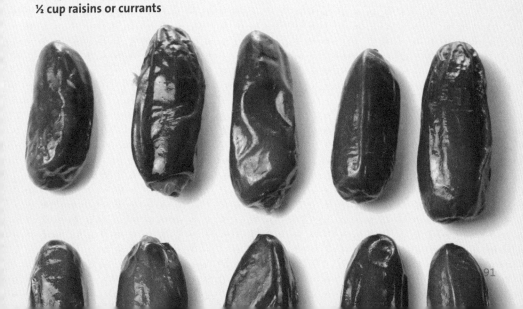

Coconut Date Bonbons and Oranges

Impress your friends with this easy-to-make snack or dessert. The miso adds friendly bacteria (or probiotics), depth in flavor, and saltiness. If you don't have miso, just add a pinch more of salt. Grated orange rind, or zest, adds a nice citrus note. We frequently make bonbons in our classes at Bastyr University where I teach because the students love them! They're easy to carry in backpacks and make a stellar post-game snack.

¾ cup pecans
1 orange
½ cup pitted dates, chopped
Pinch of sea salt
¼ teaspoon cinnamon
1 teaspoon white miso
1 tablespoon maple syrup
¼ cup shredded coconut

▶ Preheat oven to 300°F.
▶ Place pecans on cookie sheet. Toast 10 minutes, or until they give off a nutty aroma. Let cool.
▶ Zest and peel orange. Divide into wedges.
▶ Combine nuts, zest, dates, salt, cinnamon, miso and maple syrup in food processor. Pulse until texture is mealy.
▶ With moist hands, roll mixture into 1-inch balls.
▶ Spread coconut on plate. Roll balls in coconut, covering evenly.
▶ Pack bonbons and orange wedges in separate containers. Eat them together.

PREP TIME: 20 minutes
MAKES: 8 bonbons
Vegetarian, Gluten-free

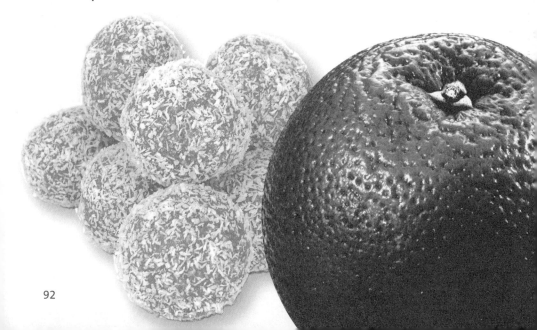

Gingerbread Molasses Cookies and Pears

Teff is a whole grain used in Ethiopia to create injera— the stretchy daily bread eaten with stews and salads. Adding teff flour makes these cookies really chewy and high in iron. Also containing iron-rich molasses, these cookies offer a double hit of this important mineral. Pears are the perfect whole fruit accompaniment.

1 cup + 2 tablespoons
  whole wheat pastry flour
4 tablespoons teff flour
1 teaspoon baking soda
½ teaspoon salt
1 teaspoon cinnamon
¼ teaspoon allspice
¼ teaspoon cloves
¼ teaspoon cardamom
¼ pound unsalted
  butter, room temperature
¾ cup brown sugar or sucanat
  (dehydrated whole cane sugar)
2 tablespoons blackstrap molasses
½ teaspoon vanilla
1 egg
1 tablespoon fresh ginger, grated
Pears

▸ Preheat oven to 350°F.
▸ Combine pastry flour, teff, baking soda, salt and spices. Set aside.
▸ Cream butter and sugar with mixer. Add molasses, vanilla, egg and ginger, and mix until light and fluffy.
▸ Mix in dry ingredients. If dough is still sticky, add more flour a teaspoon at a time until dough forms a ball without sticking to your hands.
▸ Roll into 1-inch balls. Place on greased cookie sheet. Bake 12 minutes.
▸ Pack whole pears with cookies.

PREP TIME: 45 minutes
MAKES: 2 dozen cookies
Vegetarian, Nut-free

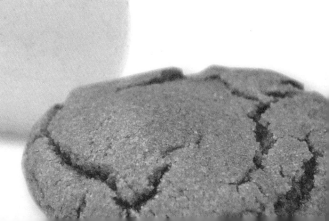

Best Spice-Kissed Oatmeal Cookies

Traditional ingredients make the best oatmeal cookies in the world. Make a bunch for the team and hand them out after the game. Be sure to use whole wheat *pastry* flour, not whole wheat bread flour, or the cookies will be too dense. Chilling the cookie dough prior to baking helps form the structure of the cookie in the hot oven before the butter melts.

1 cup butter, room temperature
1½ cups whole wheat pastry flour
3 cups rolled oats
½ teaspoon salt
½ teaspoon cinnamon
½ teaspoon cardamom
¼ teaspoon nutmeg
1 teaspoon baking soda
1 cup brown sugar or sucanat
 (dehydrated whole cane sugar)
1 cup white sugar
1 teaspoon vanilla
2 eggs
½ cup walnuts, chopped
¾ cup raisins

▸ Preheat oven to 350°F.
▸ Combine flour, oats, salt, spices and baking soda in bowl. Set aside.
▸ Cream butter, sugars and vanilla with mixer. Beat in eggs.
▸ Mix in dry ingredients. Fold in nuts and raisins.
▸ Chill dough for 30 minutes, or more if you have time.
▸ Roll into 1-inch balls. Place on greased cookie sheet. Bake 12 minutes.
▸ Remember to save some for your sports bag.

PREP TIME: 30 minutes
(plus 30 minutes chill time)
MAKES: 3 dozen cookies
Vegetarian

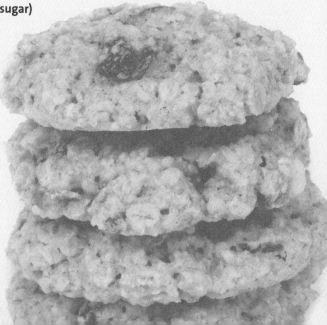

Peanut Butter Cranberry Zoom Zoom Bars

You'll love adopting these as a tried-and-true snack. They're fabulous. Hip hip hooray to colleagues Leika Suzumura and Steven Jamieson for sharing this perfect pack-in-your-sports-bag recipe with me. Add salt only if you are using unsalted peanut butter. Share them with your teammates for a better zoom zoom than any packaged protein bar.

1½ cups rolled oats
½ cup sunflower seeds
½ cup pumpkin seeds
½ cup dried coconut flakes
½ cup dried cranberries
½ cup brown rice cereal or other puffed/
    crispy whole grain cereal
⅛ teaspoon salt, optional
1 cup peanut butter or other nut butter
1 tablespoon butter
½ cup brown rice syrup
2 tablespoons honey
2 tablespoons molasses

▸ Preheat oven to 350°F.
▸ Spread oats, sunflower and pumpkin seeds on baking sheet. Toast 10 minutes, shaking every few minutes for even toasting.
▸ Add coconut. Toast 2 minutes, or until coconut turns golden. (Watch closely!) Let cool.
▸ Combine toasted mixture, cranberries and brown rice cereal in large bowl.
▸ Combine peanut butter, butter, rice syrup, honey and molasses in saucepan over medium heat. Stir until smooth.
▸ Fold into toasted mixture until evenly mixed.
▸ Plop onto greased cookie sheet. Press down with moist hands into ½-inch thick square, about 12x12 inches large.
▸ Cool completely. Pop into the refrigerator to hasten this.
▸ Cut into 2x3-inch squares. Individually wrap with waxed paper or plastic.

PREP TIME: 30 minutes
MAKES: 18 to 24 bars, depending on number of cuts
Vegetarian, Gluten-free

Tamari Roasted Nuts and Dried Apricots

Tamari-roasted nuts are a crunchy and savory addition to any backpack. Tamari and shoyu are both naturally brewed soy sauces (no chemicals, preservatives, sugar or MSG). Shoyu contains wheat, soybeans, water and salt. Tamari is wheat-free.

1 cup raw almonds, whole
1 cup raw cashews, whole
1 tablespoon tamari
   (naturally brewed soy sauce)
½ teaspoon cumin, ground
½ teaspoon coriander, ground
Pinch cayenne, optional
2 cups dried apricots
   or other dried fruit, diced

▶ Preheat oven to 325°F.
▶ Spread nuts on baking pan. Toast 10 minutes, or until golden, with a nutty aroma.
▶ Combine tamari and spices. Spread over toasted nuts.
▶ Return to oven and bake 8 minutes, or until completely dry.
▶ Mix in apricots after nuts are cool. Store in sealed container.

PREP TIME: 25 minutes
MAKES: 4 cups
Vegetarian, Gluten-free

Rice Cakes with Almond Butter and Melon Mélange

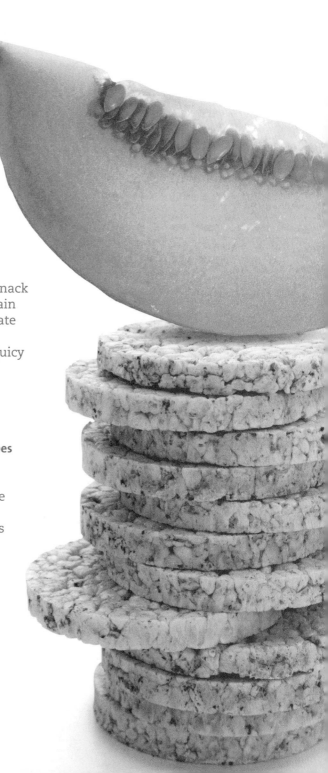

Think of this post-game snack as a triple win: whole grain rice cakes for carbohydrate refueling; almond butter for healthy protein and fats; and juicy fruits for hydration.

2 tablespoons almond butter
4 rice cakes
½ cantaloupe, bite-sized cubes
½ honeydew melon, bite-sized cubes
1 cup red grapes, halved

▶ Spread almond butter on rice cakes. Pack in container.
▶ Toss melon cubes and grapes together. Pack in container.

PREP TIME: 10 minutes
MAKES: 4 big snacks or 8 small snacks
Vegetarian, Gluten-free

Tortilla Chips and Summery Pico de Gallo

½ pound plum tomatoes,
  seeded and diced
¼ cup white onion, finely diced
¼ cup fresh cilantro, chopped
1 small jalapeño,
  seeded and finely diced
¼ teaspoon sea salt
Juice from 1 lime
5 cups tortilla chips

Fresh pico de gallo—or fresh salsa—is light years beyond the jarred version. If you prefer spicy salsa, leave the seeds in the jalapeño as you dice. It's worth paying a little extra to buy organic tortilla chips. This makes enough for a big team snack!

▶ Combine tomatoes, onion, cilantro and jalapeño in medium bowl.
▶ Add salt and lime juice.
▶ Let stand for 30 minutes before serving to allow flavors to develop.
▶ Serve with tortilla chips.

PREP TIME: 15 minutes
MAKES: 2 cups
Vegetarian, Nut-free, Gluten-free

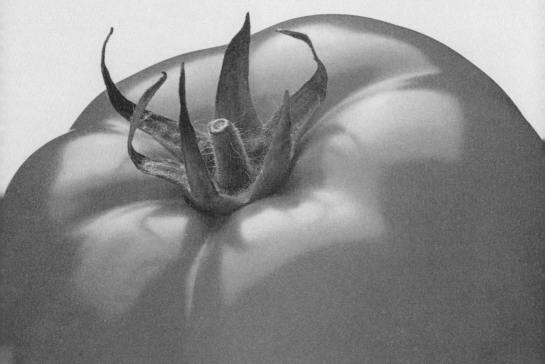

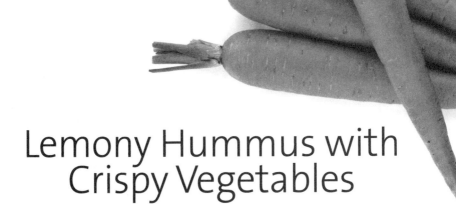

Lemony Hummus with Crispy Vegetables

Hummus is a traditional Middle Eastern spread that's delicious on vegetarian sandwiches. Grab-and-go containers of hummus and crispy veggies are also great snacks to have on hand before and after games. (Cooking note: Blanching—or flash-boiling—brings out the flavor of vegetables while preserving nutrients.)

2 lemons
2 cups chickpeas, cooked or canned
5 tablespoons tahini
   (sesame seed paste)
1 teaspoon sea salt
2 cloves garlic
3 tablespoons extra-virgin olive oil
¼ cup liquid reserved from drained beans
2 sprigs parsley, chopped
Paprika to taste
1 cup broccoli flowerets
1 cup cauliflower flowerets
1 cup carrots

▸ Bring large pot of water to boil for blanching vegetables.
▸ Zest rind of one lemon. Juice both lemons.
▸ Combine chickpeas, lemon zest, lemon juice, tahini, salt, garlic, olive oil and reserved liquid in food processor. Blend until smooth.
▸ Divide into grab-and-go containers. Garnish with chopped parsley and paprika. Can be stored in the refrigerator for up to a week.
▸ Prepare large bowl of ice-cold water.
▸ Drop vegetables into boiling water and blanch about a minute, or until color brightens. Plunge vegetables into cold water.
▸ Drain vegetables and allow to air dry. Divide into grab-and-go containers and store in refrigerator.

PREP TIME: 30 minutes
MAKES: 3 cups hummus, 3 cups blanched vegetables
Vegetarian, Nut-free, Gluten-free

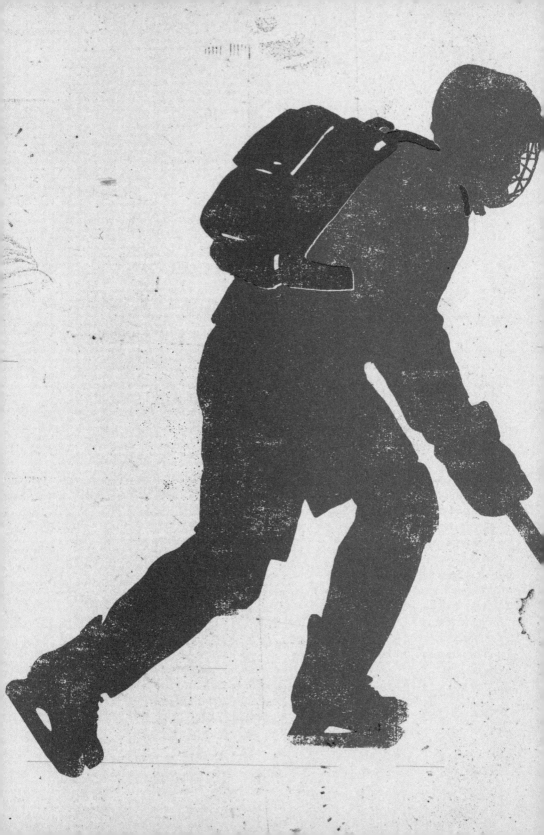

7

Pack-n-Go Snacks to Buy at the Store

Buy This

Carrot sticks and dip

Deli bean salad

Deli pasta salad

Dried fruit

Energy bars (read labels)

Fresh fruit

Fruit salad

Hard-boiled eggs

Hummus and pita

Nori rolls or inari

Toasted nuts

Tortilla chips and black bean dip

Trail mix

Turkey wraps

Whole grain sandwich

Whole grain fig bars

Whole grain muffin

Whole grain raisin bread with peanut butter

Yogurt (read labels)

Even when you don't have time to get prepared at home, you can still BE PREPARED with a short stop at the store

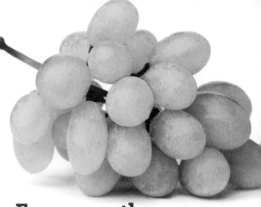

For most families with kids who play sports, time is of the essence. You don't always have the opportunity or mental space to make food at home. That's when a nearby grocery store with a deli can come to the rescue. Bring a shopping list. Avoid filling the cart with packaged convenience foods. Read ingredient lists and focus on whole foods. Shop the perimeter of the store where more whole foods can be found.

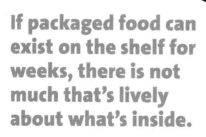

If packaged food can exist on the shelf for weeks, there is not much that's lively about what's inside.

Focus on the purpose of your purchase

Pre-game meal. You will need to combine several elements to mirror the proportions of the pre-game plate (page 41). For example, pair a sandwich from the deli with an apple from the produce department. Or, how about a deli bean or pasta salad with a variety of fresh ingredients already mixed together? Try a whole grain muffin and a hard-boiled egg for a quick pre-game breakfast. Trail mix might work when you have an early-morning game (and you've already had an excellent pre-game dinner the night before).

Mid-game snack. Buy and pack fresh, juicy fruits like oranges and grapes.

Post-game snack. Use the 4:1 carbohydrate-to-protein strategy. Pack crackers and cheese, apples and peanut butter, hummus and pita, carrots and dip, or tortilla chips and salsa. Vegetarian brown rice sushi makes a tasty post-game bite or try whole grain fig bars if you have a taste for a little sweet rather than savory.

Energy Bars: Read labels carefully and consider your purpose

My colleague, Liz Kirk, Ph.D., in the Department of Nutrition and Exercise Science at Bastyr University, offers the following advice regarding energy bars: "If you're an athlete and you're training for a competition, then you have a different purpose from someone who just wants a snack. Choose your best bar accordingly."

The good news is that there are some fantastic bars out there made with whole foods ingredients. Read ingredient labels so you know what you are eating.

To fuel activity. If you are in need of quick energy, seek out bars with high carbohydrate content (20 grams or more). Consider the source of the carbohydrates as well. Is it whole food ingredients or isolates? Select bars with fewer than 18 grams of sugar—meaning that sugar or a form of sugar (words that end in the letters -ose) is not the first ingredient. Also, make sure the bar has fewer than 15 grams of protein for quicker digestion.

To fuel recovery. The best formula for recovery is a bar with a 4:1 ratio of carbohydrates to protein. You may need to bring your calculator to the store to make sure the bar you're choosing will replace glycogen stores efficiently.

To satisfy hunger. When you are not preparing for games or practice, it's okay to choose bars with a more balanced ratio of protein to carbohydrates. Protein and fat slow down digestion and prolong fullness. And remember that fiber slows digestion as well, helping to create a more sustained release of energy.

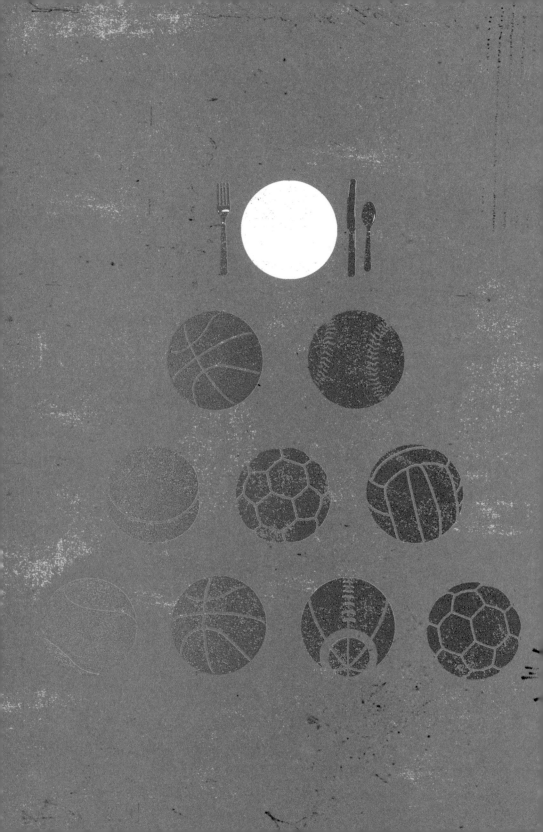

CHAPTER 8

Winning Pre-Game Meals

Make This

110% Chicken Noodle Soup

Big Mo Minestrone

Mediterranean Lentil, Sweet Potato and Spinach Stew

Chickpea Broccoli Indian Curry

Chipotle Black Bean Stew

Baja Fish Tacos and Lime Slaw

Chicken Vegetable Teriyaki

Edamame Tofu Salad

Samurai Salmon and Avocado Bowl

Hoppin' John and Chicken Apple Sausage

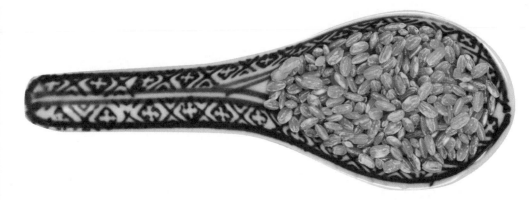

The following meals use the pre-game plate guidelines and are inspired by flavors from around the world

Many cultures depend on inexpensive carbohydrates such as rice, corn and bread to make up the bulk of the meal, while meat and other higher-priced proteins are served as flavoring or smaller sides. This meal strategy, designed to save money as well as other resources, works perfectly to fuel athletes.

You may notice that we don't use beef and pork in our recipes. These meats are fine on non-game days or off-season. But on game days, they're too heavy and slow to digest. Consider buying 100% grass-fed beef, which is lower in fat and calories, four times higher in vitamin E, and has two to four times more omega-3 fatty acids than meat from grain-fed animals.

Using your favorite recipes, compose your meals with the right proportions for better performance.

Make sure the base of the meal, the largest proportion of food, comes from whole grains and/or starchy vegetables such as sweet potatoes or lentils.

This approach ensures that quick-converting carbohydrates will give you the muscle glycogen you needed to play your best. Include protein, but relegate it to side-dish status. Always include lots of vegetables and fruits. These add the vital nutrients that transform other foods into energy while adding color, flavor and not many calories.

Cooking is fun! Players should help prepare meals whenever possible

Investing time in preparation elevates appreciation for the food. The trend in quick recipes (often with fewer than five ingredients) short-changes the flavors and colors of our meals, as well as the value we place on cooking and eating together. Perhaps one family member could make the main dish, and you can make the sides. Or vice-versa.

Don't be discouraged by the number of ingredients in these recipes. Unlike long ingredient lists on packaged foods—usually representing fillers, preservatives and marketing lingo—the ingredients in these pre-game meal recipes offer wholesome nutrition and delicious flavors. Please improvise freely! Season dishes to your family's taste. Add more spices, herbs and vegetables or skip an ingredient you don't have on hand.

Videos that demonstrate how to prepare many of the recipes in this book can be found at my online cooking program, *www.cookus.tv*.

Don't
be
afraid
to

IMPROVISE!

110% Chicken Noodle Soup

Serve with whole grain bread and basil pesto butter

Simple and delicious, this soup was a favorite in our team's pre-game meal survey. I use chicken breasts to make stock. However, you can buy pre-made stock or use any pre-baked or roasted chicken you have on hand. Any size noodle works, but my favorite is organic ribbons. Consider doubling or tripling the recipe for the basil pesto butter to freeze and use later. I use a tablespoon of pesto in Big Mo Minestrone when fresh basil is not available. To make pesto pasta, use one cup of pesto sauce for one pound of cooked pasta.

Chicken stock:
2 tablespoons extra-virgin olive oil
1 tablespoon butter
2 carrots, diced
2 stalks celery, diced
1 leek, chopped
1 onion, chopped
1 turnip, chopped
2 teaspoons salt
3 quarts water
2 bay leaves
4 sprigs rosemary
4 sprigs marjoram
4 sprigs thyme
½ cup parsley, chopped
½ pound chicken breasts (or other parts)
1 tablespoon rice vinegar

▸ Heat oil and butter in soup pot. Add carrots, celery, leek, onion, turnip and salt. Sauté until vegetables are tender.
▸ Add water, herbs, chicken and vinegar. Bring to low boil, reduce to simmer, and cover and cook 30 minutes.
▸ Remove breasts. Set aside.
▸ Strain stock and store in glass jars in refrigerator. It will keep for at least a week.
▸ Use to cook rice, simmer vegetables, thin out sauces and make super soups.

PREP TIME: 1 hour
MAKES: 3 quarts stock
Nut-free, Gluten-free

Soup:

1 tablespoon butter
1 onion, chopped
1 clove garlic, minced
1 carrot, diced
1 stalk celery, diced
5 leaves bok choy
1½ quarts chicken stock
1½ cups chicken, cooked and cut into
  bite-sized pieces
2 cups noodles, cooked
2 tablespoons fresh rosemary, chopped
2 tablespoons fresh marjoram, chopped
2 tablespoons fresh parsley, chopped
Salt and pepper to taste

▸ Heat butter in soup pot. Add
  onion and garlic. Sauté until soft.
▸ Add carrot and celery. Continue
  sautéing.
▸ Cut white stems of bok choy into
  ½-inch pieces. Roll dark green
  part of leaves and slice into thin
  strips. Set aside.
▸ Add bok choy stems, stock,
  chicken and noodles to pot. Bring
  to low boil, and then turn heat off.
▸ Add fresh herbs and bok choy
  ribbons. Cover and let sit 15
  minutes.
▸ Add salt and freshly ground
  pepper to bring out flavor.

PREP TIME: 30 minutes
MAKES: 6 big bowls of soup
Nut-free

Basil pesto butter:

1 cup basil leaves, de-stemmed,
  rinsed and spun dry
¼ cup extra-virgin olive oil
1 tablespoon pine nuts or walnuts
2 cloves garlic, peeled
¼ teaspoon salt
3 tablespoons grated Parmesan
  or pecorino cheese

▸ Combine basil, olive oil, nuts,
  garlic and salt in food processor.
  Blend until smooth.
▸ Mix in cheese to finish the pesto
  butter. Serve on warmed whole
  grain bread alongside soup.
▸ If you are making extra pesto,
  pour into lightly oiled muffin
  tins. Place in freezer for 1 hour.
  Remove frozen disks and place
  in bags. Store in freezer.

PREP TIME: 10 minutes
MAKES: about ½ cup
Vegetarian, Gluten-free

Big Mo Minestrone

Serve with Buttermilk Honey Cornbread (page 90)

Minestrone means "big soup" in Italian, and there are as many variations of this soup as there are cooks. I've used some of the classic minestrone vegetables, but my friend Elena says you can add any vegetable your heart desires. Serve this with plenty of freshly grated Parmesan and hearty cornbread.

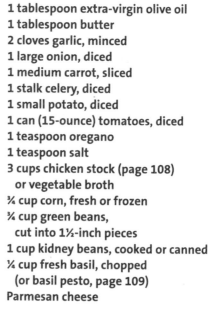

1 tablespoon extra-virgin olive oil
1 tablespoon butter
2 cloves garlic, minced
1 large onion, diced
1 medium carrot, sliced
1 stalk celery, diced
1 small potato, diced
1 can (15-ounce) tomatoes, diced
1 teaspoon oregano
1 teaspoon salt
3 cups chicken stock (page 108)
  or vegetable broth
¾ cup corn, fresh or frozen
¾ cup green beans,
  cut into 1½-inch pieces
1 cup kidney beans, cooked or canned
¼ cup fresh basil, chopped
  (or basil pesto, page 109)
Parmesan cheese

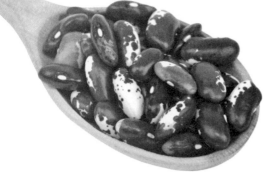

▸ Add olive oil, butter, garlic and onion to soup pot. Sauté until onion is soft.
▸ Add carrots, celery and potato. Sauté 5 minutes more.
▸ Add tomatoes, oregano, salt and stock. When soup begins to simmer, cover and cook 30 minutes.
▸ Add corn, green beans and kidney beans. Simmer 8 minutes, or until green beans are tender.
▸ Stir in fresh basil or basil pesto and black pepper to taste.
▸ Serve with freshly grated Parmesan on top and cornbread on the side.

PREP TIME: 1 hour
MAKES: 4 servings
Vegetarian option, Nut-free, Gluten-free

Mediterranean Lentil, Sweet Potato and Spinach Stew

Serve with warm pita and mint yogurt topping

Five of our favorite whole foods are all in one recipe! This stew is bursting with nutritional richness. I prefer the small, charcoal-colored French lentils. Fresh herbs always add full flavor, but substituting dried herbs is just fine, too. Buy whole wheat pita to add whole grain goodness to this meal.

2 tablespoons extra-virgin olive oil
1 onion, chopped
2 cloves garlic, minced
1 medium sweet potato, cubed (about 2 cups)
1 cup lentils
4 cups chicken stock (page 108) or vegetable stock
8 ounces tomato sauce
2 teaspoons sea salt
1 tablespoon butter
2 tablespoons fresh sage, minced
2 teaspoons fresh thyme, minced
4 cups spinach leaves, de-stemmed and chopped (about 4 ounces)
1/3 cup currants or raisins
1 teaspoon balsamic or red wine vinegar
Fresh ground pepper

▸ Heat olive oil in large soup pot. Add onion and garlic. Sauté until golden.
▸ Add sweet potato, lentils, stock, tomato sauce and salt, stirring gently.
▸ Bring to low boil, reduce to simmer, cover and cook 45 minutes, or until lentils and sweet potato are tender.
▸ Add butter, sage, thyme and currants to skillet. Sauté until fragrant.
▸ Add spinach and 2 teaspoons water. Cover and let spinach wilt for 1-2 minutes.
▸ Preheat oven to 300° F. Warm pita in covered dish for 10 minutes.
▸ When you're ready to serve, add spinach, herbs, vinegar and black pepper to stew. Serve with yogurt topping and pita bread on the side.

PREP TIME: 1 hour
MAKES: 6 servings
Vegetarian option, Nut-free, Gluten-free

Mint yogurt topping:
½ cup plain whole milk Greek yogurt
2 tablespoons fresh mint, chopped

▸ Combine yogurt and mint in small bowl.

PREP TIME: 5 minutes
MAKES: ½ cup
Vegetarian, Nut-free, Gluten-free

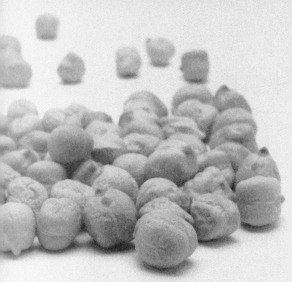

Chickpea Broccoli Indian Curry

Serve over quinoa with raita yogurt topping

Quinoa works beautifully as a bed for curries and stews. Try grinding whole cumin and coriander in a spice mill to deepen the flavor. The raita is an excellent dip for roasted potatoes (page 82).

Curry:

2 teaspoons ghee (clarified butter) or extra-virgin olive oil
1 onion, chopped
1 clove garlic, minced
½ teaspoon sea salt
2 teaspoons cumin, ground
1 teaspoon coriander, ground
1 teaspoon turmeric
½ teaspoon cinnamon
Pinch of cayenne
1 small potato, diced
1 carrot, sliced
1 cup tomato sauce
½ cup chicken stock (page 108) or water
1 cup broccoli florets
1 cup chickpeas, cooked or canned

▸ Heat ghee or olive oil in soup pot. Add onion, garlic and salt. Sauté until onion is soft.
▸ Add cumin, coriander, turmeric, cinnamon and cayenne. Sauté until bright and fragrant.
▸ Add potatoes, carrots, tomato sauce and chicken stock (or water), stirring well.
▸ Bring to low boil, reduce to simmer, cover and cook 30 minutes or until potatoes and carrots are tender.
▸ Add broccoli and chickpeas, stirring gently. Cover and cook a few minutes until broccoli is bright green.
▸ Serve over quinoa and garnish with raita.

PREP TIME: 50 minutes
MAKES: 4 servings
Vegetarian option, Nut-free, Gluten-free

Quinoa:

1 cup quinoa
Pinch of sea salt
1¼ cups water

▸ Add quinoa, salt and water to 2-quart pot. Bring to low boil, reduce to simmer, cover and cook for 15 minutes, or until all the water is absorbed.
▸ Remove lid and let rest for 10 minutes.
▸ Fluff with fork before serving.

PREP TIME: 20 minutes
MAKES: 2½ to 3 cups
Vegetarian, Nut-free, Gluten-free

Raita yogurt topping:

1 cup plain whole milk yogurt
1 teaspoon fresh mint, minced
½ teaspoon cumin, ground
Pinch of cayenne
Salt and pepper to taste
½ cucumber, peeled and seeded

▸ Combine yogurt, mint, cumin and cayenne in small bowl.
▸ Dice or grate cucumber to the texture you would like the topping to have. Squeeze excess water from cucumber and add to yogurt mixture.
▸ Add salt and pepper to taste. If you have time, chill for 20 minutes before serving.

PREP TIME: 10 minutes
MAKES: 1 cup
Vegetarian, Nut-free, Gluten-free

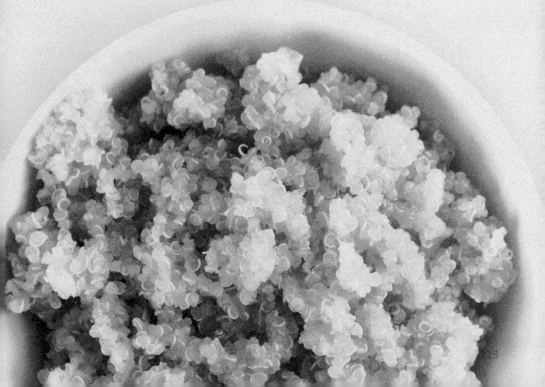

Chipotle Black Bean Stew

Serve with Grace's One-Touch Quesadillas

Mexican seasoning blends come in bulk or in spice bottles at the grocery store, usually as a combination of cumin, oregano, peppers and other spices that give a Southwestern flavor to dishes. Cooking dried, bulk beans tastes the best and is easy with a little planning. Using a pressure cooker cuts the cooking time in half. Substituting two 15-ounce cans of beans works in a pinch. Beans and tortillas will give you all the protein and carbohydrates you need to play a great game.

Stew:
1 cup dried black beans, soaked overnight (or 2 cans, 15-ounces each)
1 teaspoon extra-virgin olive oil
1 onion, chopped
2 cloves garlic, minced
1 teaspoon cumin, ground
2 teaspoons Mexican seasoning
1 dried chipotle chili
2 cups chicken stock (page 108) or vegetable stock
1 teaspoon sea salt
½ cup corn kernels, fresh or frozen
½ cup tomatoes, chopped
¼ cup cilantro, chopped
Lime
Sour cream, optional

▸ Soak dried beans overnight in 3 cups water.
▸ Heat oil in soup pot. Add onion, garlic, cumin and Mexican seasoning. Sauté until onions are soft and spices are fragrant.
▸ Add drained beans, chipotle chili and stock. Bring to low boil, reduce to simmer, cover and cook 1 hour, or until beans are tender.
▸ Stir in corn, tomatoes and cilantro, and salt to taste. Serve garnished with a squeeze of lime and dollop of sour cream.

PREP TIME: 1½ hours (plus overnight soaking)
MAKES: 4 to 6 cups
Vegetarian option, Nut-free, Gluten-free

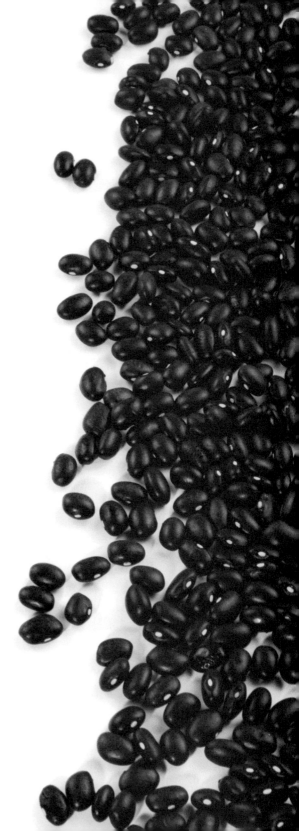

Grace's One-Touch quesadillas:
1 cup filling (any combination of
   ingredients listed below)
2 cups cheese, grated
   (cheddar, jack, mozzarella)
4 teaspoons butter
4 whole grain flour tortillas
Pico de gallo (page 98)

Filling suggestions:
Avocado, sliced
Jalapeños, finely diced
Cilantro, chopped
Tomatoes, chopped
Scallions, chopped
Onions and green peppers,
   sliced and sautéed
Roasted red pepper
Grilled chicken strips

▸ Assemble 1 cup filling, add
   2 cups grated cheese, and
   toss together.
▸ Add 1 teaspoon butter to skillet
   over low heat. Place tortilla on
   skillet and spread 1½ cups
   filling-cheese mix evenly on top.
▸ Place second tortilla on top of
   filling, press down, cover and
   cook a few minutes.
▸ Remove cover. Flip quesadilla to
   other side, press down, cover and
   cook another minute. Repeat
   with remaining tortillas.
▸ Cut 2 quesadillas in quarters to
   make 8. Serve with pico de gallo
   (page 98) or other dipping sauce.

PREP TIME: 15 minutes
MAKES: 2 quesadillas
Vegetarian, Nut-free

Baja Fish Tacos and Lime Slaw

Serve with creamy cilantro sauce

These are just like the yummy tacos you can get at restaurants, only better—the fish isn't deep-fried and the ingredients are fresh. The trick to flakey fish is not to overcook it. Remove from oven before fish is done, as it will continue to cook. Make plenty of tacos, since they're so good. Use gluten-free Tamari if you want to avoid gluten.

2 tablespoons lime juice
3 tablespoons extra-virgin olive oil
1 tablespoon tamari
  (naturally brewed soy sauce)
1 pound halibut
  (true cod or other white fish)
½ cup cabbage, shredded
4 leaves romaine, shredded
1 carrot, grated
¼ cup red onion, chopped
1 teaspoon sugar
Salt and pepper to taste
8 corn tortillas
Cheese, grated (cheddar, jack, mozzarella)
Pico de gallo (page 98)

▸ Preheat oven to 400°F.
▸ Combine 1 tablespoon each lime juice, olive oil and tamari in small bowl. Pour over fish, and marinate 30 minutes.
▸ Combine cabbage, romaine, carrot and onion. Dress with 1 tablespoon each olive oil and lime juice, 1 teaspoon sugar, then salt and pepper to taste. Set aside.
▸ Add remaining olive oil to ovenproof skillet over medium-high heat until sizzling. Sear halibut for 1 minute on each side.
▸ Place in oven and bake 7 minutes, or until fish is almost cooked through. Divide into bite-sized pieces.
▸ Place tortillas in covered pan in warm oven.
▸ To assemble tacos, put a few fish pieces in tortillas, top with lime slaw, and drizzle on cilantro sauce. Add grated cheese and pico de gallo (page 98) if desired.

PREP TIME: 45 minutes
MAKES: 8 tacos
Nut-free, Gluten-free option

Creamy cilantro sauce:
¼ cup plain yogurt or mayonnaise
1 tablespoon lime juice
2 tablespoons cilantro, chopped
1 clove garlic, pressed
¼ teaspoon cumin, powder
1 tablespoon water

▸ Whisk all ingredients for cilantro sauce in small bowl until smooth.

PREP TIME: 5 minutes
MAKES: ⅓ cup sauce
Vegetarian, Nut-free, Gluten-free

Chicken Vegetable Teriyaki

Serve with brown rice (page 79)

Sweet and salty teriyaki is always a crowd pleaser, and its good with any combination of vegetables. Marinate chicken overnight, and you'll have an almost-ready meal waiting for you the next evening. Serve this delicious dish heaped atop a mound of brown rice. It's the perfect mix of carbohydrates, vitamin-rich vegetables and protein to fuel the body for the next day's competition or practice. Use gluten-free tamari if you are on a gluten-free diet.

¼ cup tamari (naturally brewed soy sauce)
1 teaspoon fresh ginger, grated
2 tablespoons honey
1 tablespoon brown sugar
1 clove garlic, minced
½ cup water
1 pound chicken breasts, boneless and skinless
½ head cabbage, shredded
1 carrot, sliced at diagonal
½ medium onion, cubed
2 tablespoons safflower or peanut oil
2 teaspoons arrowroot (gluten-free equivalent to cornstarch)

▸ Combine tamari, ginger, honey, sugar, garlic and water in saucepan over low heat. Stir until sugar dissolves. Set aside.
▸ Cut chicken breasts into small strips, and marinate with ⅓ cup teriyaki sauce in refrigerator for up to 8 hours.
▸ Add 1 tablespoon oil to wok or skillet over medium-high. Stir-fry vegetables until bright and crisp. Set aside.
▸ Add remaining oil to wok. Stir-fry chicken until cooked through but still tender.
▸ Mix arrowroot into remaining teriyaki sauce. Add to chicken. Stir-fry over high heat until sauce has thickened.
▸ Add cooked vegetables. Stir-fry to mix flavors. Serve over rice.

PREP TIME: 30 minutes (plus 8 hours marinating)
MAKES: 6 servings
Nut-free, Gluten-free option

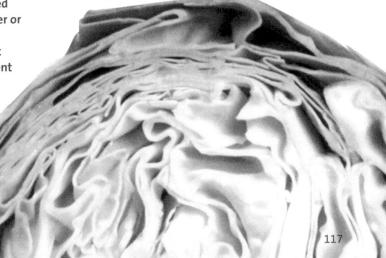

Edamame Tofu Salad

Serve buffet style with sesame chili dressing

For team meals, we like to serve a variety of foods on a big platter and allow players to make their own plates. This Asian-inspired salad is a beautiful platter of delicious and nutritious choices. Soba noodles are Japanese noodles made from gluten-free buckwheat flour. Get a head start by boiling two pots of water—a larger pot for the soba noodles and a smaller one for the edamame. Marinating tofu for a couple of hours deepens the flavors but is not necessary. Use gluten-free tamari to make this recipe gluten-free.

2 tablespoons tamari
  (naturally brewed soy sauce)
½ teaspoon fresh ginger, grated
1 clove garlic, minced
2 tablespoons water
1 pound firm tofu, cubed
4 ounces soba noodles
¼ cup toasted sesame seeds
1 tablespoon coconut oil or other
  high heat vegetable oil
1 cup shelled edamame, fresh or frozen
1 cup cabbage, shredded
1 carrot, grated

▶ Mix tamari, ginger, garlic and water in large bowl. Add tofu and marinate.
▶ Cook soba noodles in boiling water about 7 minutes. Drain noodles and mix in 2 table- spoons dressing and sesame seeds. Set aside.
▶ Pat tofu dry with paper towel.
▶ Add oil to skillet over high heat. Carefully add the tofu in and fry a few seconds on each side until browned. Drain on paper towel.
▶ Cook edamame in boiling water for 3 minutes. Strain and run cold water over it until cool. Set aside.
▶ Arrange noodles, tofu, edamame, cabbage and carrots in separate piles on a large serving platter. Put dressing in a small pitcher. Dig in!

PREP TIME: 40 minutes
(plus time to marinate)
MAKES: 4 servings
Vegetarian, Nut-free, Gluten-free option

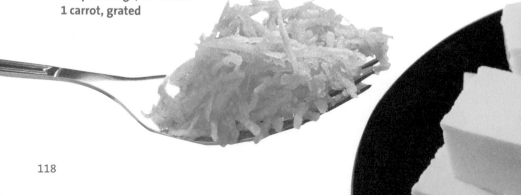

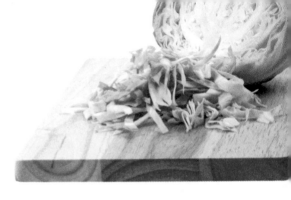

Sesame chili dressing:

2 tablespoons tamari
  (naturally brewed soy sauce)
2 tablespoons apple cider vinegar
2 cloves garlic, minced
5 teaspoons sugar
2 tablespoons mirin (or sake)
1 teaspoon ginger, grated
2 teaspoons Thai chili sauce
¼ cup extra-virgin olive oil
2 tablespoons sesame oil

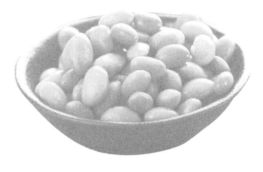

▶ Mix ingredients, except oils, in small bowl. Slowly drizzle in the olive oil and sesame oil, whisking well to emulsify.

PREP TIME: 5 minutes
MAKES: ¾ cup dressing
Vegetarian, Nut-free, Gluten-free option

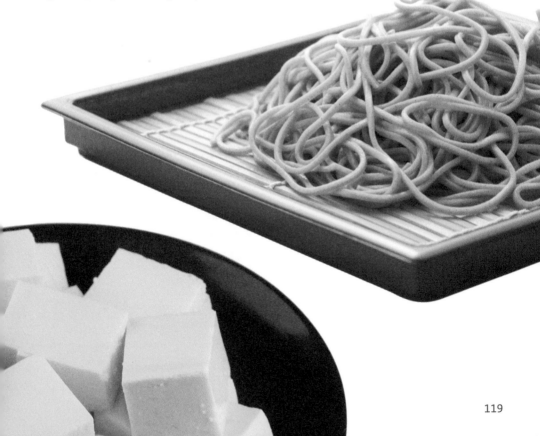

119

Samurai Salmon and Avocado Bowl

Serve with wasabi dressing and brown rice (page 79) or soba noodles (page 118)

This recipe is great for team meals since the fun part is artfully assembling your own bowl with your favorite vegetables. Getting together to chop, slice, grate and snip the vegetables is fun, too. Eating this magnificent bowl of food will give you game power. Dine and conquer!

1 pound fresh sockeye salmon
¼ cup sesame seeds
Salt and pepper
1 cucumber, sliced
2 avocados, sliced
½ daikon, grated (about ½ cup)
½ sheet nori, cut into thin strips
   with scissors
1 tablespoon coconut oil or other
   high heat vegetable oil

▸ Put salmon in shallow pan. Drizzle on 2 tablespoons of dressing, and marinate 30 minutes or more.
▸ Preheat oven to 400°F.
▸ Toast sesame seeds in dry skillet over medium heat, shaking constantly until golden and fragrant. Set aside.
▸ Add vegetable oil to ovenproof skillet over high heat until sizzling. Sear salmon for 1 minute on each side.
▸ Place in oven and bake for 6 minutes, or until fish is almost cooked through. Divide into strips. Salt and pepper to taste.
▸ Place a generous bed of rice in bowl, top with salmon strips, cucumber, avocado, daikon and nori. Drizzle dressing and sprinkle toasted sesame seeds.

PREP TIME: 45 minutes
MAKES: 4 servings
Vegetarian, Nut-free, Gluten-free

Wasabi dressing:
¼ cup sesame oil
2 teaspoons toasted sesame oil
¼ cup rice vinegar
¼ cup sugar
¼ cup tamari
   (naturally brewed soy sauce)
3 teaspoons prepared wasabi

▸ Whisk all ingredients until emulsified.

PREP TIME: 5 minutes
MAKES: over 1 cup
Vegetarian, Nut-free, Gluten-free

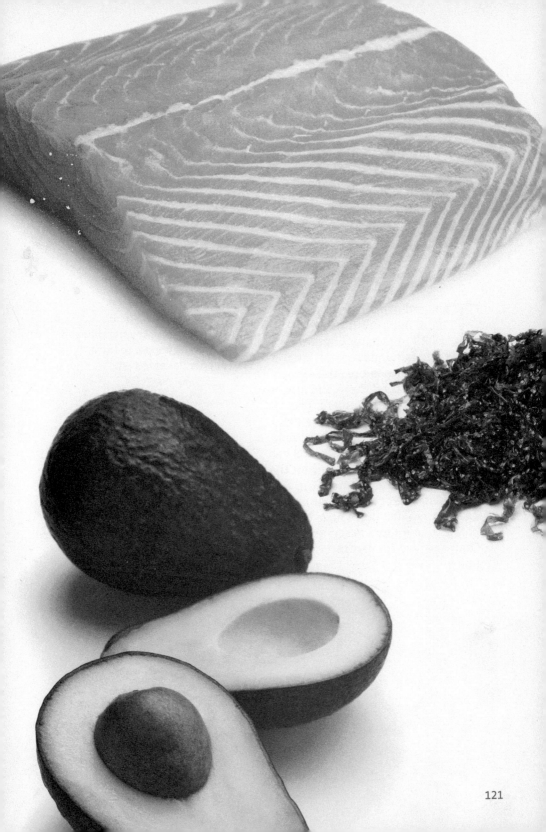

Hoppin' John and Chicken Apple Sausage

Serve with cheesy polenta

The red pepper is what makes John hoppin'! Time and planning are required to make this fabulous meal. Soak the beans the night before. And yes, you have to just stand there and stir the polenta for 30 minutes. The goal is to achieve a smooth, thick and creamy consistency. Leftover polenta with a brush of olive oil can be reheated in the broiler or on the grill for a quick and satisfying breakfast. Use brown rice or quinoa on days you just don't have the patience or energy to stir and stir. Omit sausage for vegetarians. Enjoy!

1 cup dried black-eyed peas, soaked overnight
1 sprig fresh thyme
1 bay leaf
1 squeezed orange plus water to make 1½ cups liquid
½ teaspoon sea salt
¼ cup sherry (or water)
2 links chicken apple sausage
1 tablespoon olive oil or butter
1 onion, chopped
5 cloves garlic, minced
½ red bell pepper, diced
1 carrot, sliced
½ cup corn, fresh or frozen
½ cup tomatoes, chopped
1 tablespoon fresh thyme, chopped
Salt and black pepper to taste
Red pepper flakes to taste

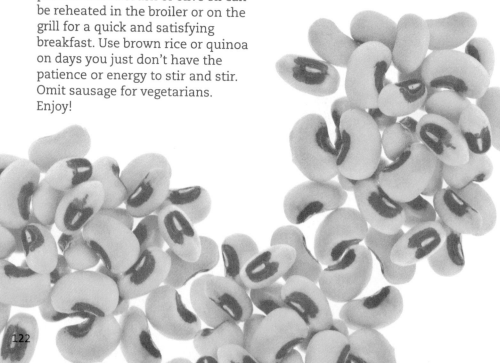

- Put drained peas, thyme, bay leaf and orange juice in pot. Bring to low boil, reduce to simmer, cover and cook 30 minutes, or until peas are tender and liquid is absorbed.
- Discard herbs, add sea salt and mix gently. Set aside.
- Add sherry or water to skillet over medium-high heat. Add sausage, reduce to simmer, cover and cook until liquid has thickened (but not blackened!).
- Uncover and brown sausages on all sides. Set aside. Slice when cool.
- Heat oil or butter in clean skillet. Add onion and garlic. Sauté until onion is soft.
- Add red pepper, carrot, corn and tomatoes. Sauté until carrots are tender.
- Add thyme, salt, black pepper and red pepper flakes to taste.
- Add cooked black-eyed peas and sliced sausage, stirring gently until flavors deepen together. Taste and adjust seasonings.

PREP TIME: 50 minutes
MAKES: 4 servings
Vegetarian option, Nut-free, Gluten-free

Cheesy polenta:
2 cups chicken stock (page 108) or vegetable stock
3 cups water
1 teaspoon salt
1 tablespoon + 2 teaspoons extra-virgin olive oil or butter
1 cup polenta (coarsely ground cornmeal)
4 tablespoons asiago or pecorino cheese
Extra-virgin olive oil to garnish

- Bring stock and water to boil. Add salt and 1 tablespoon oil or butter, and slowly stir in polenta.
- Lower heat and continue stirring 30 minutes. Adjust heat to maintain soft puckering of polenta. Stir in 4 tablespoons cheese. Set aside.
- Pour polenta into lightly oiled 8x8-inch baking dish. Smooth out top. Cool to room temperature before slicing. Serve on the side with a bowl of Hoppin' John.

PREP TIME: 40 minutes (plus cooling time)
MAKES: 8 slices
Vegetarian option, Nut-free, Gluten-free

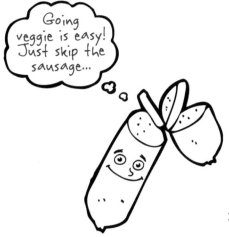

123

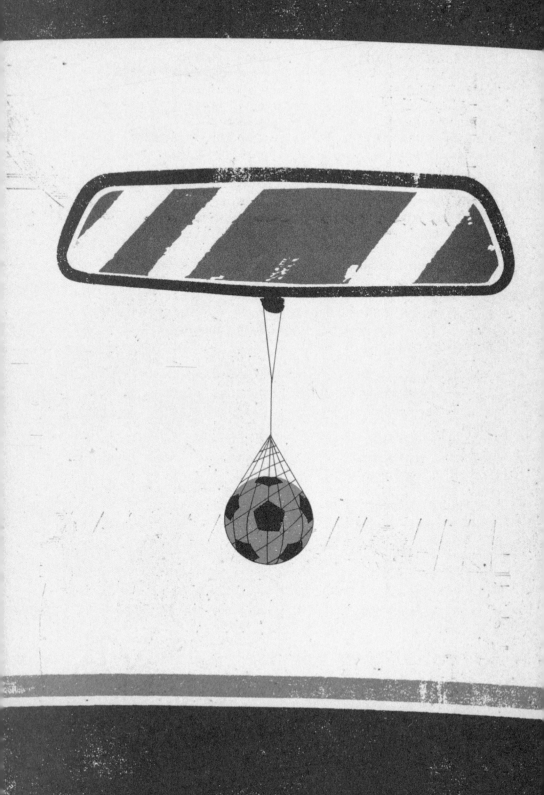

9

Food **on** the Road

Order This

Think way outside the bun. Use your phone apps. Find that locally owned ethnic restaurant. Typically, ethnic meals offer the opportunity to "make your plate" with the right proportion of nutrients.

Chinese

Ethiopian

Greek

Indian

Italian

Japanese

Mexican

Northern U.S.

Southern U.S.

Thai

Ignoring the demands of travel can put the whole team's performance at risk

My daughter, Grace, had two things that put her at an advantage for travelling to away games—cooking skills and a rice cooker. In the sleepy early-morning while finding cleats and shin guards to pack, she would also sauté whatever vegetables she had handy, add some cooked rice, and pack the food in a container to throw in her bag.

While the other players were eating paltry sandwiches provided to the team, she would whip out her fried rice and listen to the "Ooohhh. That looks so good!" from other players. I admired Grace for her resourcefulness, but couldn't help wonder why there wasn't plenty of food on the bus for everyone.

When you ride for long hours on a bus or plane, the body goes into a lethargic mode. Not only do muscles get sleepy and brains get foggy, but the body also gets dehydrated. Kids are often expected to jump off the bus, do a quick warm up and then play their best. This simply is not going to happen if the quality and timing of eating and drinking have not been considered.

PLAN WHAT, WHEN AND WHERE YOU WILL EAT AND DRINK

before travel

Eat a substantial pre-game meal before boarding the bus or car.

Bring fresh fruit to eat during the ride and a sandwich for the return trip.

FOR TRAVEL under 2 hours

Keep your water bottle out and sip, sip, sip.

Stop after the first hour and jog a few laps to keep muscles awake and digestion progressing.

FOR TRAVEL over 2 hours

All of the above and...

Plan to eat a pre-game plate two to three hours before the start of a game or event.

If you need to stop and eat, then the question is ... what and where?

My daughter played on a select team for many years. At least once or twice a season we had to drive over the Cascade Mountains to the eastern part of Washington State. During one trip we found a sweet little Indian restaurant in a small town. The food was good—plenty of fragrant rice and tasty vegetables. We bookmarked the spot. From then on it was our routine watering hole going east.

Too often the assumption is that young people will only eat "kids' food," meaning poor-quality fast food.

Cost is usually a factor as well. The default food for traveling teams seems to be cheap pizza and sodas. There are better choices.

Choose food venues based on the best food for players. Let everyone know that this is part of the game plan. Want better performance?

Think outside the bun. Don't necessarily look for the nearest chain restaurant or convenience store. Use your phone apps. Find that locally-owned ethnic restaurant. Typical ethnic meals offer the opportunity to "make your plate" with the right proportion of nutrients.

Find a good ethnic restaurant and have fun ordering

When we think about the proportions of the pre-game plate (page 41) carbohydrates in the form of whole grains are front and center, with fresh fruits, vegetables and some protein as teammates.

This is the proportion of many ethnic meals since traditional cultures throughout the ages depended on affordable carbohydrates to provide the majority of calories for their meals. Italians have pasta. Asians depend on rice. Masa is part of Central American meals.

Fruits and vegetables are eaten seasonally, and meats are used in moderation, often as flavoring rather than center plate.

Many of the recipes for pre-game meals we included here are inspired by ethnic foods and flavors. Players can try these new tastes out at home first to gain more confidence ordering at an ethnic restaurant.

3

THREE BIG REASONS FOR ATHLETES TO CHOOSE ETHNIC FOODS

They **provide** a substantial proportion of grains and vegetables for efficient production of muscle energy.

They **expand** the food repertoire and exercise the taste buds of young athletes. Plus, eating with peers can persuade the picky eaters to try new foods.

They **encourage** eating lower on the food chain. Animal proteins tend to be used more sparingly in ethnic cuisines. Better for the body, better for the planet.

Find a good grocery store

Most grocery stores these days have well-stocked delis and prepared foods to order. You can pick up some oranges and apples along with a deli bean salad. If your team is at an out-of-town tournament for a few days, scout out a good grocery store and stock up on some of the foods in the Pack-n-Go to Buy from a Store list (page 101).

❗ Don't under-estimate the power of a snack

One Sunday afternoon, about two hours from home, our team was surprised by a win that meant we were sticking around for a championship game. There were about two hours to kill before the final—not enough time to go to a restaurant. We knew the girls needed some food to replenish before the championship game. I drove around and finally just stopped at a grocery store. I bought a loaf of raisin bread and some oranges, and dashed back to the field where the girls were waiting. This was a very inexpensive and effective snack. I don't remember if the team won the game...but I do remember a happy bunch of girls sitting on a grassy hill, grabbing slices of raisin bread out of a bag.

10 ORDERING IDEAS FOR SUPERB PERFORMANCE

1 Chinese
wonton soup, vegetable mu shu, Buddha's Delight (stir fried vegetables), sesame noodles

2 Ethiopian
harira (vegetable soup), yemiser w'et (lentil stew), yetakelt w'et (vegetable stew), injera (bread)

3 Greek
spanakopeta (spinach pie), lentil soup, hummus and pita, Greek salad

4 Indian
chickpea curry, spinach paneer (cheese), vegetable biryani, mango lassi, raita, rice, naan (bread)

5 Italian
spaghetti with marinara, pesto pasta, margherita pizza, minestrone soup, garlic bread

6 Japanese
miso soup and rice, inari (rice in tofu pocket), udon noodles, sushi

7 Mexican
tortilla soup, guacamole and quesadillas, rice and beans, fish tacos, bean burrito

8 Northern U.S.
squash soup, corn bisque, vegetable stew, grilled salmon

9 Southern U.S.
cornbread, Hoppin' John, jambalaya, buttermilk biscuits, mashed potatoes, collard greens

10 Thai
Tom Ka Gai (coconut chicken soup), Pad Thai, yellow curry, fresh spring rolls

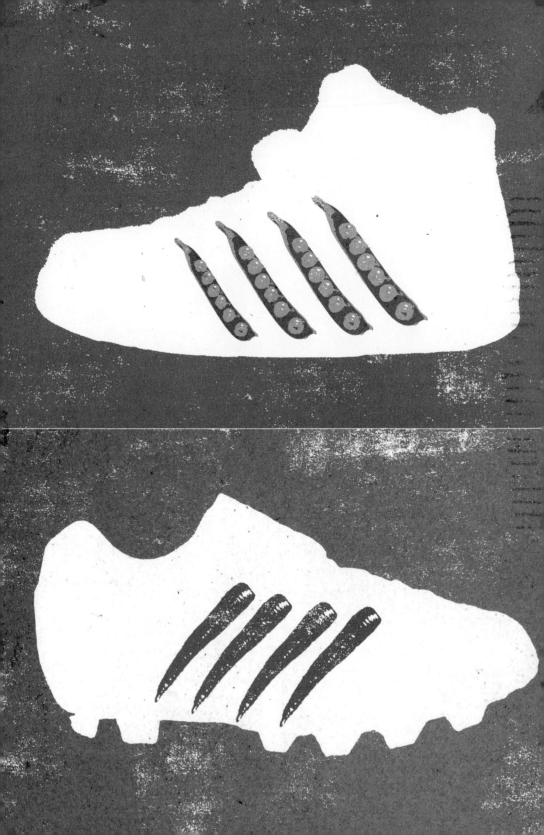

CHAPTER

10

Team Meals

Sharing a meal builds camaraderie and community

Eating is more than just taking in nutrients and easing your hunger. Eating engages us with the natural world (where food comes from, namely plants and animals). Eating together also engages us with each other when we share meals.

! Organize a team meeting around a meal

Share the pleasure of eating freshly prepared, beautifully presented foods with your teammates. Try different tastes and flavors, and compare notes about what you like. You can model good eating habits for your teammates.

! Learn cooking skills to eat better for the rest of your life

Many young people haven't learned basic cooking skills like how to cut an onion or what "simmer" means. Try a cooking class as a pre-season team-building activity. You can ask a parent or adult friend who loves to cook to be your teacher.

10 TEAM MEALS

1

Rise-Shine-and-Score Pancake Feast
Try pancakes, hash browns, scrambled eggs, toast and fresh orange juice. This is a great early morning get-together before the drive to a big game.

2

Play-Hard Pastamania
Have several families bring their favorite pasta dishes and copies of the recipes. Encourage pasta dishes that include vegetables and some form of protein. Other families can bring green salads and beverages to round out the meal.

6

The Spaghetti Advantage
Provide spaghetti and several types of add-ins—fresh vegetables, simple marinara, basil, mushrooms, cheese, olive oil, and pesto. Add warm garlic bread and a huge tossed salad to fuel up.

7

Mediterranean Match-Up
Spread out a platter of fresh tomatoes, olives, cucumbers and feta cheese. Add hummus, some herb-roasted chicken and a big casserole of spanakopita (spinach pie) for everyone to enjoy.

3 Baffle-the-Opponent Baked Potato Spread

Someone will need to bake a whole bunch of potatoes. Add all kinds of toppings like cheddar cheese, steamed broccoli, chopped scallions, fresh chives, tuna salad, sour cream and chickpeas. Get creative!

4 We-Got-Mo Mexican Fiesta

Bring tortillas, salsa, black beans, rice, cheese, olives, guacamole, grilled chicken strips, refried pinto beans, shredded lettuce dressed with lime vinaigrette— and set up a "build your own burrito" bar.

5 Take-Action Rice and Kabob

Use rice cookers to make mounds of brown rice. Have plenty of big chunks of vegetables like zucchini, portobello mushrooms, green and red peppers, and onions. Add pieces of marinated chicken breast or tofu, and make your own kabobs to grill and slide over a bed of rice.

8 Power-Up Bagels and Fruit

How about a no-cooking team meal? Lay out a variety of bagels and spreads (cream cheese, roasted bell pepper, olive tapenade, hummus). Serve the bagels with bowls of freshly sliced fruit or have a parent make a few pitchers of fresh-fruit smoothies.

9 On-Your-Mark Hot Soup and Fresh Bread

This is a homemade-soup potluck. Bring your family favorite— minestrone, black bean, mushroom, lentil, tomato, and chicken noodle. Have several loaves of fresh bread, sliced thick and warmed in the oven. There's nothing quite as nourishing and delicious as simple soup and bread.

10 Pack-n-Go Snackathon

The night before a big tournament or a final playoff, gather team members and make Pack-n-Go snacks (page 101) together to take the next day. Cut up and pack fruit for halftimes and breaks. Bake muffins and quick breads for the post-game glycogen-window chow-down.

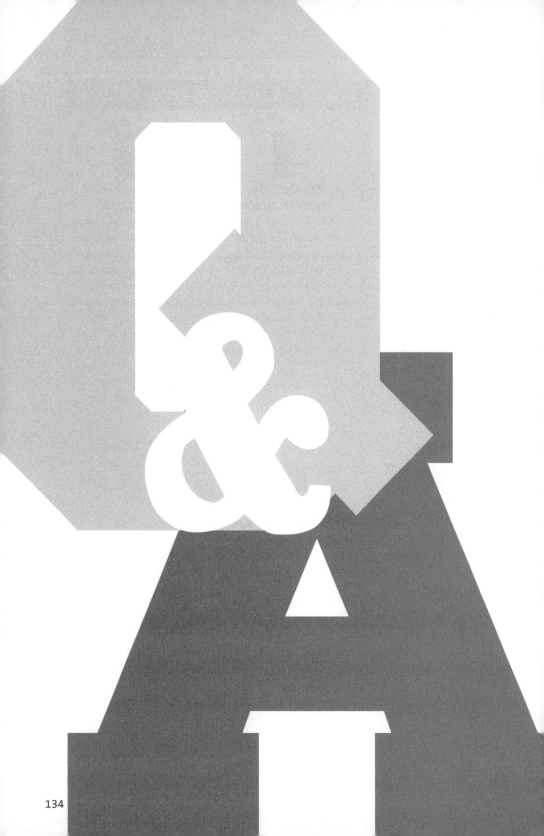

FOOD

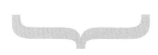

If I'm vegetarian, can I get enough protein?

No problem. A plant-based diet with ample whole grains, beans, nuts, seeds, dairy and eggs provides enough protein. Many elite athletes choose to eat a vegetarian diet. However, the cheese-pizza-and-soda-pop vegetarian is woefully lacking in nutrients. Choose whole, minimally processed foods, preferably foods you could prepare in your kitchen.

How do players on gluten-free diets get enough carbohydrates?

Eat plenty of gluten-free whole grains such as buckwheat, quinoa, rice, corn, teff, wild rice and certified gluten-free oats. These are chock-full of wholesome carbohydrates. More and more packaged crackers, breads, pastas and baking mixes are now available gluten-free.

Are organic foods better?

Food without synthetic chemicals such as pesticides and fertilizers, hormones and/or antibiotics is better for our bodies and for the planet. Research demonstrates that people who switch to an organic diet knock down the levels of pesticide byproducts in their urine by as much as 90%. At a minimum, consider following the Environmental Working Group's Shopper's Guide (www.ewg.org/foodnews/guide), which identifies the "dirty dozen" (foods that commonly have the highest levels of pesticides) and the "clean fifteen." You may be surprised to see favorite fruits and vegetables on the dirty dozen list, such as apples, strawberries, spinach, grapes and potatoes!

Should I choose low-sugar foods?

Not necessarily. Be careful of low-sugar products as they often use artificial sweeteners. When you eat these chemical sweeteners, they simulate sweetness in your mouth and the body naturally expects the carbohydrates to follow. When it doesn't, the body gets mixed messages that may cause cravings for more sugar. Studies have linked artificial sweeteners to cancers. Instead, focus on whole foods where there are no added sugars, or packaged foods where sugar is not one of the first three ingredients.

Should I be concerned with my salt intake?

The salt you add in cooking or at the table is not the real problem. If you tend to buy processed, packaged foods, then yes, it is important to be aware of your recommended allowance. Remember that sugar can mask the taste of salt. For example, soda is high in sodium but you can't taste it because there is so much sugar in the formula. Yet another reason to read labels.

PERFORMANCE

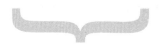

What changes will I see in my performance if I change my diet?

If you follow our guidelines and consume fresh whole foods, you will likely experience increased energy, stronger muscles, quicker decision-making, better concentration on and off the field, faster recovery, deeper sleep, clearer skin, healthy weight for your body and milder PMS if you're a female. Work *with* your body's needs instead of against them to reap these re-wards.

How do I eat for sports such as soccer, swimming or track that have several events in one day?

Eat well during the days before a daylong event. During the event day you will need to take advantage of every break for constant refueling. This means drinking and snacking (sip and nibble) at every opportunity in order to delay the rate at which you exhaust your muscle glycogen. If you haven't seized your snacking opportunities, your performance in upcoming events will suffer.

What if I have an early-morning game?

The best plan is to get up early enough to eat a substantial pre-game breakfast. If you prioritize sleep ahead of that, eat your pre-game meal the night before and have a light carbohydrate snack, such as a bagel and fruit (no heavy protein or fat), an hour before the game.

What can I do if I feel a slump in the second half?

Try eating a piece of fruit during the break. If that works for you and you feel your energy pick up, incorporate that snack into your game plan. More importantly, reflect on your current regime. Have you been eating regular meals? Resting enough? Training too hard without food and rest? Be aware of how your body is affected by your daily patterns to help avoid slumps.

What are signs and symptoms of heat exhaustion and heatstroke?

Heat-stress illnesses can range from heat rash and cramps to life threatening exhaustion and heatstroke. Heat exhaustion is characterized by hot skin with some moisture, dizziness, fainting, headache, nausea, vomiting and muscle cramps. Heatstroke is characterized by hot but often dry skin, vomiting, and central nervous system problems (such as confusion, impaired judgment, agitation, aggressiveness, apathy, and convulsions). Heatstroke requires immediate medical intervention, primarily due to high core body temperature (>105°F).

You can help prevent heat-stress illness by being aware of your environment and the extent of your exertion, and by taking steps to cool down your core body temperature. Rest periods, frequent hydration breaks, appropriate clothing, and scheduling practices during cooler times of the day can help stave off heat-related illnesses.

Is there anything I can eat to help me recover from an injury or illness?

Excess stress, lack of rest, overtraining, and subpar nutrition overtax our immune system, leading to colds, flu or infections. Eating a well-balanced diet with ample carbohydrates, nutrient-rich vegetables and adequate protein will help fuel the immune system. Limit those unhealthy food and drink choices that steal energy and vital nutrients away from the repair and recovery process.

Should female athletes be concerned about iron?

Iron deficiency is the most common nutritional deficiency, particularly in children, teens, and female athletes. Iron depletion in female athletes ranges from 13% all the way up to 80%, depending on the sport. Iron depletion progresses to iron deficiency, and finally to anemia.

So remember to include iron-rich foods in your diet, and have your iron levels checked periodically. Keep in mind that too much iron can be dangerous, so try to get your iron from foods first. Then, if needed, check with your health-care professional about supplemental iron.

IRON INTAKE BY AGE RECOMMENDED DAILY ALLOWANCE	EXAMPLES OF GOOD SOURCES OF IRON
CHILDREN 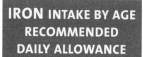 **4-8** 10 mg	**Oysters**, cooked, 3 oz — **6.1** mg
CHILDREN 9-13 8 mg	**Soybeans**, cooked, ½ cup — **4.4** mg
FEMALES 14-18 15 mg	**Pumpkin & squash seeds**, roasted, 1 oz — **4.2** mg
MALES 14-18 11 mg	**White beans**, canned, ½ cup — **3.9** mg
FEMALES 19-30 18 mg	**Blackstrap molasses**, 1 Tbsp — **3.5** mg
MALES 19-30 8 mg	**Lentils**, cooked, ½ cup — **3.3** mg

Oysters, cooked, 3 oz — **6.1** mg

Soybeans, cooked, ½ cup — **4.4** mg

Pumpkin & squash seeds, roasted, 1 oz — **4.2** mg

White beans, canned, ½ cup — **3.9** mg

Blackstrap molasses, 1 Tbsp — **3.5** mg

Lentils, cooked, ½ cup — **3.3** mg

Spinach, cooked, ½ cup — **3.2** mg

Kidney beans, cooked, ½ cup — **2.6** mg

Sardines, canned in oil, 3 oz — **2.5** mg

Chickpeas, cooked, ½ cup — **2.4** mg

Ground beef, 15% fat, cooked, 3 oz — **2.2** mg

Tomato puree, ½ cup — **2.2** mg

Cashew nuts, dry roasted, ¼ cup — **2.0** mg

Clams, 3 oz — **1.4** mg

Raisins, 1.5 oz — **0.8** mg

Source: USDA National Nutrient Database for Standard Reference 23

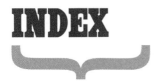

INDEX

Recipes

RESODRCES

}

We hope this list sparks your interest to learn more about sports nutrition and food.

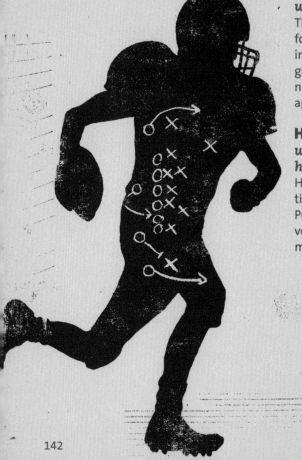

Web

Food

Cookus Interruptus
www.cookus.tv
Cynthia and company created this online cooking show to teach viewers how to cook fresh, local, organic foods despite life's interruptions. The program features more than 150 videos demonstrating ways to make super fantastic whole food dishes (including many in this book).

USDA MyPlate
www.choosemyplate.gov
The newest iteration of the USDA's food guidelines is presented as a plate instead of a pyramid. We've used this graphic to represent how to eat when not training and really appreciate the approach of this new graphic.

Healthy Eating Plate
www.health.harvard.edu/plate/
healthy-eating-plate
Harvard Health Publications and nutrition experts at the Harvard School of Public Health came up with their own version of MyPlate where they make more specific dietary recommendations.

Sports

Institute for the Study of Youth Sports
www.educ.msu.edu/ysi
This site from Michigan State University's Department of Kinesiology focuses on "the beneficial physical, psychological, and social effects" of children and youth participating in sports. As parents we sometimes get lost in the urge to have our child's team win. This site reminds us how all the other benefits of youth sports outweigh the W or L.

Let's Move
www.letsmove.gov
This is First Lady Michelle Obama's initiative to change the way kids think about food and nutrition. Exercise and good nutrition will set children on a healthier path. The site includes clear, simple steps to help parents, schools, health-care providers, community leaders, and kids achieve the goal of a healthier generation. You go, Michelle!

Moms Team
www.momsteam.com
Brooke de Lench started this site to educate viewers on a wide array of youth-sports topics from health, safety and nutrition to the psychology of parenting a young athlete. She shows how parents can make youth sports less focused on winning games and more about having fun. I've followed her site more than 10 years and it just keeps getting better and better.

Books

Feeding the Whole Family: Recipes for Babies, Young Children, and Their Parents
by Cynthia Lair
My first book, an homage to whole foods, offers close to 200 recipes. You'll find plenty of shopping guides, tips for picky eaters, and ideas on how to create balanced meals everyone will like.

Food Rules: An Eater's Manual
by Michael Pollan
This little book summarizes the whole adventure of eating with such common sense. Young people will find it easy to read, and parents and coaches will find many aha! moments.

Sundays at Moosewood Restaurant
by the Moosewood Collective
Each section of this large, attractive book encompasses a different culture. Wonder what's for dinner in Africa? The Caribbean? Maybe Japan? The recipe answers are here. Explore a different country each Sunday like they did!

What to Eat
by Marion Nestle
Ms. Nestle has become the matriarch of common sense in the nutrition and food world. Her extensive grocery-store tour, catalogued in this book, will answer all your questions about what's on the shelf and in the produce aisle.

Cynthia Lair is a certified health and nutrition counselor and author of the popular cookbook, *Feeding The Whole Family*. She is also co-creator of the humorous online cooking program, **Cookus Interruptus** (www.cookus.tv), where she combines cooking fresh, organic whole foods with improvisational theater. Videos on how to make many of the recipes in this book can be found there. Cynthia is the curriculum director of the Culinary Arts Program and core faculty member of the Nutrition and Exercise Science Department at Bastyr University. In between her teaching, writing and cooking, Cynthia has been a soccer mom for more than 14 years and remains a loyal fan of the sport. She lives in Seattle, Washington.

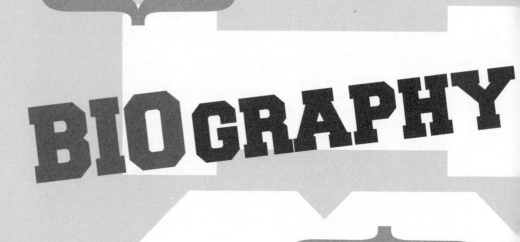

BIOGRAPHY

Dr. Scott Murdoch received his Master of Science degree in Exercise Physiology and a doctorate in Nutrition and Human Performance. He is also a Registered Dietitian. Scott has over 20 years of teaching, research, and clinical practice in human nutrition and physical performance. He has also competed in more than 90 triathlons, including three Ironman World Championships, and played tennis professionally for 18 years. He is the proud father of two athletic boys and lives in Bend, Oregon.